PRAISE for THE ROAD BACK TO ME

"When you read this book you will both be inspired and empowered. Adena has captured the essence of what it means to struggle and overcome. Her story will give you hope and her principles will leave you with the ability to move through whatever is going on in your life. A must-read for anyone who wants to truly thrive!"

— DENICE KENNEDY, DMK SOLUTIONS

"After reading hundreds of books in the self-help genre over two decades, I am rarely surprised. Adena's book is the exception! Her personal story is gripping, raw, and emotionally affecting. Anyone who has ever wondered: How can I emerge from my woundedness and live a life of freedom and authenticity, embrace my past honestly, and move toward a life of joy and fulfillment? Adena shows us a new path forward. Moreover, she educates us about the heart-wrenching, soul-depleting effects of long-term illness. For anyone who has suffered serious health problems, been misdiagnosed and misunderstood by family and friends, this book offers a fountain of water in a dry and thirsty land. In the world upside-down epoch of history we are now experiencing, Adena poses us not a sentimental, saccharine fix...but if we are willing to do the work, she illuminates how to move from darkness to light."

— GORDON MARTIN, YAMAHA EXECUTIVE CONSULTANT

"Adena is very honest and is true to herself. I felt she was speaking directly to me. Adena has a well of compassion and a very caring vibe about her, which everyone wants and needs when talking about sensitive topics."

— KELLY GOFF, SIMPLE-N-PERSONAL NOTARY

"I truly hope that if you have suffered through life in any manner with health issues, loss of a loved one, financial setbacks, relationship problems, family issues, etc. that you take the time to read this book as there is most likely something within these pages that will inspire, encourage, and elevate you in some way, shape, or form, catapulting you to the next level whether that be in knowledge, truth, experience, success, or just being able to wipe the slate clean and start life over fresh with a new canvas— as Adena mentions in her story "The Perfect Storm."

— JEREMY WILSON, WILSONWORKS CONSTRUCTION LLC

"Adena's book restored my belief in the strength and perseverance of the human spirit. It remains the most powerful force on earth. Thank you Adena!"

— KEVIN CARR, VINTAGE VEST CO.

The ROAD BACK

To Me

MY GIFT TO YOU

Thank you for purchasing *The Road Back to Me*.

Here is a link to the exclusive soundtrack:

www.AdenaSampson.com/theroadbacktomesoundtrack

I hope this moves you!

A ROADMAP TO RECOVERY AND HEALING

ROAD
The
BACK
To Me

9 PRINCIPLES FOR NAVIGATING
LIFE'S UNEXPECTED TWISTS & TURNS

ADENA SAMPSON M.Sc.

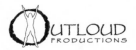

Published by Outloud Productions

Publishing Services provided by Paper Raven Books

Publisher's Cataloging-in-Publication Data

Names: Sampson, Adena, author.
Title: The road back to me : 9 principles for navigating life's unexpected twists and turns / Adena Sampson, M.Sc.
Description: "A roadmap to recovery and healing" -- from title page. | Includes bibliographical references. | Las Vegas, NV: Outloud Productions LLC, 2021.
Identifiers: LCCN: 2021908560 | ISBN: 978-1-7366910-2-1 (hardcover) | 978-1-7366910-1-4 (paperback) | 978-1-7366910-0-7 (ebook) | 978-1-7366910-3-8 (audio)
Subjects: LCSH Self-actualization (Psychology). | Resilience (Personality trait) | Success. | Conduct of life. | BISAC SELF-HELP / Personal Growth / General | SELF-HELP / Motivational & Inspirational
Classification: LCC BJ1581.2 .S26 2021 | DDC 158.1--dc23

First Printing, 2021 | Printed in the United States of America

This book is dedicated to all the outcasts, the trailblazers, the light workers, those who love fiercely, the highly sensitive ones, the bold, the brave, the courageous, and the strong.

To all those suffering long term with COVID-19, chronic Lyme disease, and any of its coinfections and cofactors such as chronic active Epstein-Barr virus, mold illness, autoimmune disorders, heavy metal toxicity, underlying genetic mutations, and any and all deemed unseen "mystery illnesses" that the medical industry has yet to fully acknowledge and understand.

This goes out to anyone healing from a broken heart, childhood trauma, codependency, and addictions, as well as their loved ones, in hopes that this will bring you closer together through awareness, education, insight, growth, empathy, compassion, and understanding.

To the stubborn ones who are suffering in silence and refusing to seek help, I pray this empowers you to become your own health advocate, saving you time, money, and any further unnecessary pain on the road to recovery.

It is my hope that this book inspires each and every one of you to take your power back, to love yourself fully, to trust your intuition, and to choose to be a part of the solution for a brighter tomorrow.

I see you, I hear you, I feel you…

"Here's to the crazy ones. The misfits. The rebels. The troublemakers. The round pegs in the square holes. The ones who see things differently. They're not fond of rules. And they have no respect for the status quo. You can quote them, disagree with them, glorify or vilify them. About the only thing you can't do is ignore them. Because they change things. They push the human race forward. And while some may see them as the crazy ones, we see genius. Because the people who are crazy enough to think they can change the world, are the ones who do."

— STEVE JOBS

CONTENTS

INTRODUCTION

"Our beliefs control our bodies, our minds, and thus our lives."
— BRUCE H. LIPTON

We are born with all this magnificence, lighthearted beings in a state of innocence, embodying pure love and joy, only to be weighed down and covered up by this false reality as we know it, forgetting who we are and where we came from. As time passes we find ourselves off track, seeking the way home, spending our whole lives working backwards trying to get back to where we started in the first place.

We spend most of our formative years, particularly during the first seven years of childhood, mimicking our parents' projected thoughts and belief patterns...the good, the bad, and the ugly! Scientific evidence suggests that aside from passing down our physical hereditary traits, we also pass down behavioral traits, survival instincts, and trauma from generation to generation within the family lineage through epigenetic mechanisms that have a direct effect on our cellular DNA and thus our overall health.

Growing up, you may have gotten the wrong impression due to hurtful projections coming from your parents, teachers, and even the kids at school. Many of us developed coping strategies while internalizing these inaccurate messages as truth. Because these belief systems were programmed into us at a very young age, they became a part of our self-image, affecting how we perceive ourselves and the world around us. This misguidance becomes the blueprint on which our psychological development takes place and often shows up in the form of self-sabotage, addictions, codependency, health issues, and more. We may lack purpose, compare ourselves, underestimate our worth, and even push people away due to a deep-seated fear of abandonment. We may find ourselves walking on eggshells, apologizing all the time, and unable to ask for help. We may feel this overwhelming responsibility to take care of others and to try to solve their problems, ultimately putting other people's needs above our own.

Too many of us spend our lives trying to fix what we feel is inherently wrong with us, because our need to belong is so deeply embedded into our biology. In an attempt to fit in, we may feel pressured to conform to societal norms, seeking outside ourselves for guidance and validation, only to be met with false projections and unmet expectations. Some of us wear many masks and play many roles. We strive for perfection in an imperfect world pretending to be someone we're not, while forgetting who we really are. We get so caught up in seeking approval that our true beauty gets lost. We hold back our most precious gifts, for fear of being judged and not accepted. We keep experiencing the same challenges over and over again and we don't understand why.

If you have been struggling for years, I want you to know that you're not alone and that it's not your fault. Our culture has been lying to you. We live in a time where sensitivity, compassion, vulnerability, and kindness are desperately needed yet greatly undervalued. We have become an industrialized, isolated society that capitalizes on convincing you that something about you is not good enough. It's a broken system! It's been designed to keep you coming back over and over again, only to leave you feeling defeated and hopeless, unworthy and broken, like there is something missing.

Let us cut right through the illusion. It's time to expose the lies that we've been telling ourselves that have prevented us from living life full out. The question is: Can you handle the truth? It's important that we recognize the presence of love in a world gone crazy with fear, dig in and remember the truth in the face of illusions, and uncover our true selves in a time and space that feeds us false advertising and fake news. The truth is, there is nothing "wrong" with you and there is no "fixing" required. The only thing we need to be saved from is our own beliefs about ourselves and others. All that's required is a shift in perspective: the realization that who you are right here, right now, is enough!

That being said, there is no magic pill or quick fix when it comes to healing our trauma. True transformation is about becoming aware of the habits and behaviors that are holding you back and are keeping you stuck in unhealthy repeating patterns. It's about taking responsibility, understanding your triggers, and becoming conscious of your beliefs and the choices you make. The first step is to gain awareness as to how these patterns are playing out and repeating in our lives and then deciding to make a change to break the cycle. The moment we choose to change our perception is the moment we rewrite our story.

My journey began long before I even came into the picture; generational disturbances run deep within my family circuit, impulses so strong they have echoed on. Even though I don't remember much from my childhood, I vividly recall looking up at a black-and-white picture that hung on my grandmother's wall depicting my grandparents' wedding in "Hitler's bedroom" just six months after the war had ended. A strong statement and a stark reminder of having overcome the insurmountable.

In more ways than one, it's nothing short of a miracle that I'm alive today. Out of the seven million Jews that were murdered in World War II, my grandmother was the only one in her immediate family to survive the Holocaust. The main reason she survived, we were told, was because of her beautiful singing voice. My grandfather served in the Royal Tank Corps of the British Army, fought in the Battle of the Bulge, and helped liberate the camp at Bergen-Belsen on April 15th 1945. That's how they met. Like many others, they had formed a trauma bond—a loyalty that is formed due to negative circumstances, binding people together due to a shared experience. They did their best in the years to come, although it was hard to erase the damage that had been done. Both of them witnessed and experienced atrocities that were etched into their psyches forever.

Needless to say, both my parents grew up in broken homes, and like their parents before them, their relationship was founded on unstable ground. My mother and father met in middle school and started dating right out of high school. Because of their tumultuous upbringings—which included witnessing compulsive behaviors and both of their parents filing for divorce in a time when it was unheard of, leaving them feeling devastated—they had formed a similar bond. At the age of twenty-one—throwing caution to the wind—my father asked my mother to marry him just two weeks before moving to the Orient for work. Two years later, I was born.

As you can imagine, my entrance into this world was filled with adventure, just like the rest of my life has been. Never a dull moment! My parents—young and still figuring out who they were—did the very best they could to give me and my sisters all that they never had, and yet despite their well-intended efforts, none of us were left unscathed.

Many of the beliefs that were inherited from our family of origin were adopted to protect us, to help us survive. However, over time, these core beliefs can turn into limiting beliefs that no longer serve us. If there's a place within us that feels in any way, shape, or form unworthy of love, we will draw experiences to us to validate that belief.

In the pages to follow, I will be sharing my story—one of excruciating heartbreak, severe chronic illness, and financial devastation—a twelve-year journey that had me fighting for my life. This journey brought with it much pain, and yet yielded many gifts. Somewhere along the way, I realized that I had created some of these problematic dynamics and perpetual experiences due to my unconscious core beliefs. I learned through pain that the love I was seeking externally was within me. When it came down to life or death, many times over, the only choice I had was to choose me. What saved my life was the decision to fully love and care for myself. I realized that I could no longer continue to give from an empty cup, leaving myself drained and void of energy—my life force completely depleted. I had to live in my truth, learn how to say no, and take time out to recharge my own batteries. In order to fully heal I had to take my power back, strengthen my mindset, explore my limiting beliefs, and move past them to understand that things were not happening *to* me, they were happening *for* me—especially when everything I knew came crashing down, was torn apart, and swept away. I had to be willing to walk blindly in faith, trust my inner knowing, persevere, and commit to doing whatever it took to overcome, irrelevant of my circumstances.

Your decision to read this book tells me that you've hit a wall of some sort that is forcing you to take a look at your life from a different perspective. Your current circumstances have left you doubting yourself and questioning your own sanity. You may be feeling overwhelmed, stressed, anxious, depressed, scared, tired, angry, confused, disheartened, alone. You're at a crossroad. You're uncertain, things are unclear. Perhaps you got laid off, maybe you've lost your business and you're having to pivot to make a change in your career. Perhaps you're going through a breakup or a divorce and you're having a hard time with the transition. Maybe a loved one has passed on and you're having a tough time coping with it. Perhaps you're an empty nester, now unsure of what to do with yourself and wondering what comes next. Maybe you're dealing with a health issue that has stopped you dead in your tracks.

This book is for you if you've been feeling stuck, if you've been searching aimlessly for answers and solutions and are unsure of how to move forward. This book is for those of you who have been through hell and back and are looking to remember the truth of who it is you are. This book is for those of you who are ready to take a good look in the mirror and question your core beliefs: what you were taught, what you were told.

Suffering serves a purpose, for it signals the need for change, and the pain we are now experiencing is telling us that we must change our ways. It's time to reevaluate the way we live. We need to remember what our true source is. Where our support and sustainability really come from. For the truth is we are provided for in every moment, even when it looks otherwise. Every cloud has a silver lining, which means no matter how bad a situation may seem, there's always a bright side—if we choose to see it. Difficult times are like dark clouds that pass overhead and block the sun. When we look closely at the edges of every cloud, we can see the sun shining through.

A miracle is a shift in perspective, and that's exactly what I've been given. My hope is to give you hope, no matter what you are going through right now. Whether you are sick, losing your job, a loved one, or even the roof over your head, I want you to know you are not alone. You have the courage inside you to move through this. If I can do it, you can too!

I promise you, if you read this book through till the end, you or someone you know and love will benefit greatly from reading it. The road back to self is a journey. On this journey, you're going to discover that you hold beliefs that aren't even your own. You're going to uncover your authentic self and unlock your true potential. You're going to apply nine principles that will change the course of your life. These principles are a roadmap to recovery and healing, for anyone fighting a battle to withstand the storm.

Within these principles, I offer up concepts, daily practices, and exercises to help you navigate life's unexpected twists and turns that, when put to use, will give you the strength you need to shift your perspective, push past your comfort zone, face your fears, reclaim your power, and turn everyday challenges into victories.

You will be given the opportunity to reevaluate how you measure success—to understand the driving force behind the self-sabotaging thoughts and behaviors that are holding you back. You will develop and instill new empowering habits and beliefs that will improve the quality of your life, creating a new paradigm rooted in authenticity. You will be given the tools you need to build a stronger sense of rapport, confidence, and trust in yourself and in all your relationships. You will learn how to ask for help, expanding your vision of what is possible and increasing your capacity to receive. You will get the support you need to forgive, to let go of grief, to feel compassion, gratitude, and love for others, no matter how they may have hurt you in the past. You will have the chance to rekindle the joy in your life and ignite your passion, to rediscover yourself, to redefine your identity, and to align with your true essence, your true purpose. You will gain resilience—the ability to bounce back—the courage to rise and the clarity you need to move forward. Overall, you will experience a newfound freedom, bridging the gap between where you are and where you're meant to be—a happier, healthier, more empowered you!

Life is short. Can you really afford to stay stuck, unhappy, and unhealthy much longer? Now more than ever, the world needs you to rise up and reclaim your power. No more dimming your light to make others comfortable. It's time to break free from the chains that bind. You were born with an unbreakable spirit that wants to be unleashed. So let us rise to the occasion and take the opportunity to start over with a clean slate. Learn how to live in your truth and express your true colors. Paint a new picture of the life that represents the truth of who you are. Let it all hang out and let your light shine through.

PART I

THE PERFECT STORM

"Once the storm is over, you won't remember how you made it through, how you managed to survive. You won't even be sure, whether the storm is really over. But one thing is certain. When you come out of the storm, you won't be the same person who walked in. That's what this storm's all about."
— HARUKI MURAKAMI

This is not a tale of one specific event in my life that has changed me…but rather a culmination of events, stressors, and triggers that created a domino effect—The Perfect Storm.

MY STORY

*"Our greatest glory is not in never falling but in rising
every time we fall."*
— Confucius

E very circumstance presents an opportunity for growth. The
question is, how far are you willing to go? How deep are you
willing to go to find your true essence?

I was on an upward spiral throughout my life; my passion
and commitment to being of service attracted incredible
opportunities and a community of great friends. Then, in 2008,
everything changed. Everything just fell apart—my health, my
relationship, my finances—my world came crashing down and
so did I!

I had managed to acquire a resistant strain of staph, otherwise
known as MRSA, in my lymph nodes and right breast tissue that
had relapsed for the second time, leaving me in critical condition.
Four nurses tried to stick me with an intravenous seven different

times before it finally took. I lay there thinking, "God? Is there something you're trying to tell me?" The message rung out loud and clear: How many times do you have to be pricked before you bleed? When was I going to draw the line and let go of this relationship that no longer served me? When was enough, enough? Was I willing to die for it?

They say love is blind, and I would have to concur. My higher self and intuition had been trying to get my attention from the very beginning. I had been walking on eggshells for far too long, and I was sick and tired of not being seen, heard, or understood. I had unconsciously hooked into an unhealthy dysfunctional pattern that was being repeatedly played out, and by sticking around, I kept the cycle alive.

Part of me was in denial, afraid to let go, afraid that if I did I'd be making a big mistake. And that's when it happened. As I lay there with a PICC line in my arm, heavily drugged, my partner threw another one of his weekly fits and walked out. For me, this was the last straw! At the time, I was numb. It seemed almost impossible to deal with the immense pain in my heart in addition to all the pain I was feeling in my physical body. I felt abandoned and devastated, deprived of comfort by the very man who claimed he wanted to be my husband. For when it mattered the most—in what seemed to be my weakest moment, my darkest hour—he wasn't there.

I was on the floor gut-wrenched; I felt broken, my wings tattered and torn. I felt like I was dying inside, and in a way I was. There were days I couldn't get out of bed. I would wake up many mornings with an empty pit in my stomach feeling like I was going to hurl. I was angry at myself for not trusting myself, my intuition, and all the signs. I felt like a fool. I was hurt, left questioning and trying to renegotiate with the universe. Why, God? Why did I feel so close yet so far away from the man I loved with every inch of my being and breadth of my soul? There must be some mistake. I somehow felt conned, like I had been wronged, baited with a beautiful, shiny, red, juicy apple only to find after taking a bite that it had been poisoned.

I found myself in a scary place, a place where fear resides. A place where I had somehow, even for just a moment, forgotten what having faith was. I felt tired and overwhelmed, so far removed from myself, and I just couldn't seem to find my way home.

The Great Imitator

"Things are not always what they seem; the first appearance deceives many; the intelligence of a few perceives what has been carefully hidden."
— PHAEDRUS

Spending most of my days in bed, I was slow to progress. Aside from the staph infection, it became clear that I had been exposed to black mold, left dealing with the dangers of mold toxicity and systemic candida. My adrenal glands were shot, liver inflamed, hormones a mess, and in addition, I had a bad case of chronic fatigue and fibromyalgia. Daily debilitating symptoms included, but were not limited to: full body aches, joint pain, brain fog, memory loss, migraines, waking feeling hungover, fever, night sweats, hot flashes, red itchy eyes, postnasal drip, sore throat, swollen glands, nausea, diarrhea, edema, low blood pressure, light-headedness, shortness of breath, chest pain, heart palpitations, insomnia, extreme fatigue, dark circles under the eyes, low libido, and more.

Days turned into weeks, weeks into months, and months to years. I went from doctor to doctor, took test after test, and had treatment after treatment. I was in and out of the hospital, prescribed excessive amounts of medications, and racked up thousands of dollars in debt. I was misdiagnosed again and again, having to jump through hoops in a flawed system to find the answers and get the care that I so desperately needed.

Due to lack of research funding—coupled with unreliable diagnostic testing and false negatives—I suffered for years before I was diagnosed with chronic Lyme disease in January 2015.

Did you know that Lyme disease is the most common, fastest growing vector-borne illness nationwide? It currently affects 300,000 people a year in the United States alone; this number is an estimate and does not reflect all the cases unaccounted for, as most cases go unreported. To give you some perspective, Lyme disease is more prevalent than hepatitis, breast cancer, and HIV combined.

It's no wonder Lyme disease is deemed the "great imitator," as it can mimic the symptoms of some 350 different diseases, including but not limited to: multiple sclerosis (MS), Alzheimer's, and bipolar disorder. Because of some of the unrecognized aspects of this insidious epidemic in the mainstream medical field, Lyme disease has become increasingly challenging to diagnose. Not everyone gets the "classic" bull's-eye rash, and many don't recall being bitten.

Contrary to popular belief, ticks that transmit Lyme disease are not limited to northeastern wooded and grassy environments. They can be seen in every state across the country and around the globe—whether that be in a desert landscape or your backyard. Birds migrate them and deer, horses, dogs, squirrels, and mice carry them. We often think that ticks are easy to spot, although at the nymphal stage, they are as small as a poppy seed and can go virtually undetected.

Many people are also under the assumption that the only way to acquire Lyme disease is from a tick bite. In addition to transmission by ticks, Lyme disease may also be transmitted by sand fleas and mosquitos through fluid exchange during intercourse and via any route by which blood or tissue from an infected host may enter the body, i.e. transfusions, transplants, and through the placenta from mother to child during birth.

Another widely misunderstood aspect of Lyme disease is that taking a simple course of oral antibiotics should do the trick. The Centers for Disease Control and Prevention states, "people treated with appropriate antibiotics in the early stages of Lyme disease usually recover rapidly and completely." This statement leads you to believe that Lyme disease is easy to treat and that most cases can be cured with a two-to-four-week standard antibiotic regimen. This couldn't be further from the truth! Hence why chronic Lyme disease—also known as post-treatment Lyme disease syndrome (PTLDS)—has become a highly controversial medical term.

This is a multisystem disease that can affect virtually every tissue and every organ in the human body. The bacteria that causes Lyme disease is a corkscrew-shaped bacteria that is known to bury itself deep within its host's tissues and organs. That being said, the use of antibiotics inhibits the replication of bacteria, primarily addressing the bloodstream, and does not directly kill and eradicate the bacteria in other areas of the body where the stealthy pathogen hides—including the cyst-like and biofilm forms that are antibiotic resistant. This is why it's typical to experience going in and out of some sort of remission-like state only to find it short lived and followed by a so-called relapse as the residual persister cell bacteria shape shift and recirculate, repeating the cycle all over again.

The Long and Winding Road

"The definition of insanity is doing the same thing over and over again and expecting different results."
— ALBERT EINSTEIN

You would think one would get excited after being properly diagnosed—as you could then better address the problem at hand and be more streamlined in your approach. However, treating chronic Lyme disease and its coinfections is not a straightforward task, but rather far more complex.

It is well known that Lyme disease is caused by the spirochete bacterium *Borrelia burgdorferi*. What isn't as well known is that different strains of bacteria, viruses, protozoan parasites, and fungi can be transmitted as well. Some of the coinfections that I harbored included babesiosis, *Bartonella, Mycoplasma, Chlamydia pneumoniae, Rickettsia,* and *Powassan* virus. The severe immune dysfunction caused by these tick-borne infections also allowed for other opportunistic infections such as Epstein-Barr virus (EBV), cytomegalovirus, and HHV-6 to flourish.

As you can see, Lyme disease is not one disease, but rather multifaceted in nature due to the many cofactors involved. For example, being exposed to mold or having a genetic predisposition that makes one more susceptible to mold-related illness are often overlooked factors in chronic Lyme disease as well as in other conditions such as rheumatoid arthritis, Crohn's disease, cancer, and more. Mold spores release mycotoxins that damage the immune system and make one more sensitive to bacterial endotoxins, hence further exacerbating overall symptoms. Both have an effect on the immune system and make the other more difficult to treat.

The same goes for EBV, which suggests other cofactors involved and a multi-microbe link. It has been linked to several autoimmune diseases such as Sjogren's, lupus, and most thyroid disorders where system disrupters—like high viral loads—contribute to chronic immune dysfunction. Some believe chronic active EBV is the main cause and reason behind several debilitating mystery illnesses.

Did you know that approximately 95% of the world's population is infected with EBV? EBV is known to spread from person-to-person through bodily fluids, primarily saliva. Transmission is impossible to prevent, as even symptom-free people carry the virus. You may be more familiar with the term *mono*, otherwise known as the "kissing disease." Mono is just one form of EBV, which usually stays in its dormant state once you've had it. After you've had it, the antibodies will show as having had a past infection. Functional medicine does not yet fully understand the gravity of EBV—as they are still unable to test and treat it effectively—hence why it's easy to misdiagnose and hard to address.

People with compromised immune systems aren't able to control the infection, allowing the virus to reactivate and remain active—linger and wreak havoc—instead of going into its latent (inactive) phase. Similar to the stealthy nature of Lyme, it's easy for this virus to hide and at times go undetected in the bloodstream. It lies dormant in our tissues and organs, commonly in the liver and spleen, waiting for an opportunistic time to get triggered and reactivated. This happens when immune functions become depressed in times of high stress.

There are various stress factors that can trigger EBV. They normally come in the form of a loss or a major life change, such as the death of a loved one, going through a hard breakup, loss of work, lack of finances, frequently having to move, etc. I experienced every single one of these stressors and triggers— which kept compiling—never giving me a chance to breathe and fully recover.

It's All In Your Head

"Two roads diverged in a wood, and I—I took the one less traveled by, and that has made all the difference."
— ROBERT FROST

Healing is not a one-size-fits-all course, but rather an individual one. Up until this point, a Band-Aid approach was used instead of getting down to the root of the problem. I was an anomaly to all the doctors. What was working for many other patients wasn't working for me. On almost every lab test, I seemed to have a slightly elevated white blood count that the doctors would completely disregard. The immune markers that tend to be low in chronic Lyme patients were low, and my inflammation markers were off the charts! To top it off, the doctors missed my thyroid issue time and time again due to the way they were ordering and interpreting the tests.

Western medicine wasn't cutting it, so I turned to integrative medicine—alternative therapies and doctors who were thinking outside of the box—using cutting-edge research and treatments to help heal patients. Live blood analysis showed an excessive amount of free radical damage and oxidative stress, high uric acid levels, and a handful of different bacterial, yeast, fungal, and parasitized microorganisms. Treatments included ultraviolet blood irradiation (UBI) and ozone therapy, intravenous hydrogen peroxide and vitamin C drips, glutathione pushes, hyperbaric oxygen therapy (HBOT), osteopathic and chiropractic medicine, immunotherapy, homeopathy, acupuncture, advanced cellular therapy, hypnosis, CranioBiotic technique and the use of magnets, microcurrent technology including biofeedback and the Rife machine, quantum healing, infrared saunas, colonics, ionic foot baths, Epsom salt baths, bioidentical hormone replacement therapy (BHRT), low dose naltrexone (LDN), and more.

At one point, I was on a protocol that consisted of managing to remember to take up to forty different supplements, hormones, and medications—multiple times a day—while adhering to a strict low-carb, celiac-friendly, lectin-free diet: no gluten, no dairy, no grains, no legumes, no sugar. I was spending roughly $30,000 a year—that I didn't have—in out-of-pocket medical expenses that insurance wouldn't cover. Leaving no stone left unturned, I was willing to do whatever it took to get the proper care I needed. Little did I know, I was beginning yet another journey down the rabbit hole.

It's helpful to imagine a stagnant pool of water—hard to clean unless it's irrigated first. Eventually. the body becomes overloaded with toxins and its natural detox mechanisms become sluggish. To add to this, those of us that have an underlying MTHFR gene mutation issue (yes, you read that right)—otherwise known to some of us as "the motherfucker gene"—are unable to methylate and detox fast enough in order for our body to efficiently eliminate toxins, thus creating a toxic body burden. *As a side note: You can be sure we will be discussing the importance of having a sense of humor in Principle #6: Lighten Up.*

Methylation is a biochemical process that plays an integral role in almost all of our bodily functions, controlling everything from our stress response to our immune response, and from our brain chemistry to our metabolism. For example, a deficiency of methylfolate in our body lowers glutathione levels—glutathione is known as the "master antioxidant"—and low levels lead to toxin buildup in the bloodstream and tissues. Also, you could be lacking certain vital nutrients, vitamins, and minerals that help create the proper amounts of methylfolate that your body needs for energy, as poor methylation leads to imbalanced homocysteine levels.

Problems with methylation are not always genetic in nature, as there are numerous things that can disturb the methylation pathway. For example, exposure to the heavy metals mercury, lead, arsenic, aluminum, and cadmium is pretty common in today's world, and the buildup of this heavy metal toxicity in our system brings added stress to the methylation cycle. Also, some researchers believe—for those suffering with Lyme—that *Borrelia* organisms and other microbes feed on magnesium, thus depleting magnesium levels and reducing your ability to methylate.

It is also known that Lyme disease can contribute to the accumulation of ammonia in the body, thus hindering the body's ability to remove ammonia. As pathogens are killed off in the body, causing ammonia levels to spike—creating more toxicity—it's not uncommon to have an inflammatory die-off reaction called a Herxheimer reaction. This temporary worsening of symptoms is an indication that the treatment is working. However, one can have a hard time separating the symptoms of the disease itself from the Herx reaction, a.k.a. "cytokine storm." You may already be familiar with this term, especially in news related to the coronavirus— linked to what is now known as "COVID-19 long-haulers." A cytokine storm, simply put, is when the immune system goes into overdrive.

This so-called healing crisis had me in a 24/7 pain cycle that was never ending. Looking back at pictures of myself over the last decade, it's clear to see that I was completely out of body and glassy-eyed. I was experiencing symptoms of depersonalization, depression, anxiety, panic attacks, and cognitive impairment—living with daily brain fog, difficulty finding words, slowness of recall, and incorrect associations—as well as short-term and long-term memory issues and other debilitating neurological symptoms, which included brain swelling and atrophy of the frontal lobes.

Along with this came extreme irritability and bouts of "Lyme rage" that would seem to come out of nowhere. This phenomenon has little to do with the moral character of the person experiencing it, but rather with the manifestations of Lyme disease, its coinfections, and the impact they have on the central nervous system. A study in neuropsychiatric disease found that 68% of people suffering from Lyme and associated disorders experienced explosive anger and homicidal or suicidal thoughts.

In these overwhelming outbursts of anger, I felt out of control and helpless. I found that the remnants of my high-functioning self was judging my feelings about the circumstances at hand, beating myself up about the episodes, and measuring myself by unreasonable standards and expectations. I was being too hard on myself by thinking, "I should know better." I caught myself apologizing for my behavior, as if the way I was "being" was unacceptable, not good enough in some way. I was my own worst enemy. I felt forsaken, betrayed by life, having no solid or stable ground to stand on. My spirit was crushed and left grieving. I wasn't thriving, living, or even surviving; I was merely existing. Call it a "dark night of the soul," if you will—a complete collapse.

I came close to dying many times over from the complications of this horrific disease. Forced into isolation, I was unable to do the simplest of tasks, and having to choose to do just one thing on any given day took all the energy I had. I was no longer able to make plans and keep up with the pressure of being present at social functions. It was all dependent on how I would feel that day. I missed out on so much: every business opportunity, holiday celebration, and birthday party. I was forced into a situation that gave me no choice but to learn how to choose me, over and over again.

Being told that you are attention seeking and selfish for trying to take care of yourself is inaccurate and hurtful. There is a fine line between being selfish and self-loving. It was hard not to wonder, if I had cancer instead of chronic Lyme disease, would the people around me finally grasp the severity of the situation? Would it then be deemed more acceptable to miss out on social gatherings and specific life events? Top Duke oncologist Dr. Neil Spector claims, "Lyme is the infectious disease equivalent of cancer." Due to the controversy and widespread ignorance of this life-threatening infectious disease, people don't receive the level of care and compassion that they should, and are many times left to suffer in silence.

One of the hardest things to deal with is the lack of understanding and support. There are those that would lead you to believe that you are to blame and that your illness is psychosomatic in nature; if only you could just remain positive, you could will yourself better. The psychological ramifications of being called a hypochondriac by your sister and being looked at like you're crazy by doctors who have no clue what they're doing is devastating! "How can you be so sick with nothing tangible to show from your tests and your symptoms?" It's crushing being told that this debilitating multisystemic illness is "all in your head." Enter PTSD.

It's important to find the strength within ourselves to discern fact from fiction when dealing with sick-shaming skeptics and cynics. People seem to be under the assumption that if you're feeling sick you must "look sick." Anyone who's dealing with a chronic illness has heard time and time again, "But you look great!" as if they're questioning the validity of the fact that you're literally fighting for your life! I guess when you're considered "high functioning," it can be misleading. What about the pressure felt every time a loved one asks, "how are you?" It takes too much energy to try to explain and listen to someone else's opinion of what they think you should do—like you haven't already tried everything under the sun and aren't willing to do whatever it takes. All you can muster up is, "I'm okay," all the while unable to provide them with the answer they so hopelessly crave.

The Show Must Go On

"Life is not about waiting for the storm to pass. It's about learning how to dance in the rain."
— Vivian Greene

For a handful of years—due to the neurological impact of this disease and the severity of the cognitive impairment—I was unable to continue working in sales, marketing, and consulting in the manner that I was used to. My brain was foggy and I found myself unable to communicate as clearly and efficiently as I once did. I had to figure out another way to keep myself afloat.

Music has always been a love of mine. I grew up writing songs, singing, playing the guitar, performing on stage, and spending a lot of time in the studio. Somewhere along the way, in the midst of my travels, I set it aside for a bit. Little did I know, it would all come full circle, in a time when I needed it the most.

Music literally saved my life, and I don't say that lightly. It gave me a sense of purpose, a reason to live, and a chance to shine a light in the darkness. The only time I wasn't in pain was when I was on stage for that three-to-four-hour window. It was as if all time stood still, an altered state if you will. The endorphins released probably had something to do with it, although I believe it was much more than that; it was a connection to the present moment, the only moment that was guaranteed. *We will most definitely be diving into the importance of embracing the present moment in Principle #7: Live for Today.*

What once came easy for me, however, was no longer the case. Aside from the fact that I was having a hard time remembering lyrics, I was also having recurrent issues with hoarseness that I'd never encountered in all my years of being professionally trained. As time passed, it became clear that this illness was affecting my voice too! Dr. Daniel Cameron, a nationally recognized leader for his expertise in the diagnosis and treatment of Lyme disease and other tick-borne illnesses, says, "Lyme disease is one of several infections that can cause a person to lose their voice."

If it wasn't one thing, it was another, yet my spirit kept persevering. I played through full fevers, migraines, severe nausea, and more. By the time I got home I could barely move, and sometimes, it would take me days to recover. I was tired and weary, but I never missed a gig as long as I had a voice. Like the old saying goes, the show must go on! With a smile on my face and the intention to be of service in my heart, no one would have known what was going on behind closed doors.

I've been suffering in silence, behind closed doors
Walking a wire with no end in sight
Tired and weary, it's been one hell of a ride
Trying to hide this pain inside

Wish I felt as good as everyone says I look
I'm just wearing a smile to mask the hurt
Tougher than the rest, no one knows what it's like
Trying to hide the pain inside

It's hard to believe, and even tougher to understand
A long and lonely road
My scars tell a story of life trying to break me
Fighting a battle to withstand the storm

This is not living, it's just merely existing
And I am barely hanging on
My hands are worn and my heart is torn
Trying to hide this pain inside

It's hard to believe, and even tougher to understand
A long and lonely road
My scars tell a story of life trying to break me
Fighting a battle to withstand the storm

It's hard to believe, and even tougher to understand
A long and lonely road
My scars tell a story of life trying to break me...

Tired and weary, it's been one hell of a ride
Trying to hide the pain inside
Just trying to hide this pain inside

"The Pain Inside" by Adena Sampson

Man in the Mirror

*"God grant me the serenity to accept the things I cannot change, the
courage to change the things I can, and the wisdom to know
the difference."*
— Reinhold Niebuhr

The extent of our knowledge creates our reality, because the mind
can only contemplate that which it has been exposed to, hence
the illusion. How we perceive things has to do with our beliefs.
Most of us develop our beliefs based on what we were taught at a
young age. We tend to take those beliefs and preconceived ideas
and project them on to those we love. In order to have a healthy
relationship, you need to be able to remain present to tune

into the same station, otherwise you end up on two different airwaves—and there is nothing but static.

I wasn't actively looking for another relationship while in the midst of my health crisis, although along the way, I fell into dating a bit from a place of vulnerability, seeking some joy and excitement in the moment to escape the harsh reality of my day-to-day pain. In doing so, I attracted a few players and emotionally unavailable men…until I met someone who I thought was safe, someone who I shared a deep soul connection with, who became my best friend—my greatest teacher!

They say that desire is the root to all suffering. As time went by, he longed for more than just a friendship and was unable to cast his romantic feelings aside. As much as I cherished what we shared, I knew that I wasn't able to help facilitate a conscious, co-creative partnership from the state I was in, and didn't want to risk losing the friendship we had built knowing it wouldn't be the same. I was afraid we'd end up resenting each other in the long run. Once again, my intuition was nudging me. There had always been an underlying sense that something was a little off-kilter. Was he really looking for love? Or just looking for help? As we grew closer and our bond strengthened, I found myself minimizing and rationalizing the red flags, giving into his needs and desires to be loved in that way. Let's be honest, I needed to be held too. I think a part of me was afraid that no one would love me through the ugly. The fiercely independent woman that I once knew had no choice but to ask for help and be open to receiving it.

As time went by, the dynamics of our relationship had changed, and I found myself placed in a role of being more of a parent than a partner. The man I had come to know as "love bug" was unrecognizable. My best friend who once had my back was nowhere to be found. It felt like he was purposely looking for a fight, constantly placing me on the other side of the fence. It's as if by a flick of a switch, he had short-circuited, completely checked out. I was heartbroken by his inconsistency, empty apologies, and leftover presence. The better I felt, the worse it got between us. It seemed the boundaries I set to try to break the codependency were only adding fuel to the fire, magnifying the spaces within him that never felt good enough to begin with. It was playing out just as I feared it would; our connection was slipping through my fingers and I was grasping at straws.

There is nothing more disheartening than realizing after years and years of trying to escape from your dysfunctional childhood that you are still recreating it. As human beings, we are drawn on an unconscious level towards the familiar, as familiarity breeds comfort. We tend to attract partners with different attachment styles that have the same childhood wounds as us but act them out in the opposite ways. We were playing out the typical victim/rescuer entanglement—each of us looking to fill a void—longing for the love, security, and affection we didn't receive as a child.

Both of us were raised in families where addictions existed, which meant growing up in environments that were predictably unpredictable. Oftentimes when you're not given the attention and emotional support you need during a key developmental time in your youth, you adopt certain coping mechanisms. These unhealthy dynamics and coping strategies can leave us unaware of how to get our needs met as an adult, and can have negative lasting effects that continue to be passed down generationally, until someone is willing and able to break the cycle. Research has shown that adverse childhood experiences create an elevated risk for developing a wide range of health problems across a lifetime.

I dealt with my childhood wounds differently than he had. I learned early on, due to my highly sensitive nature and empathic ways of absorbing the energy of those around me, how to cope. I could walk into a room and immediately sense tension, sadness, and any discomfort. It was hard to differentiate my feelings from those of others, and all too often, I would experience their emotional pain as my own. I felt everything and everyone. I could see things coming from miles away, and somehow I got the idea that it was my responsibility to fix it and make things right.

As the eldest of three, I carried the burden of feeling the weight of the world on my shoulders. I never really felt heard or witnessed as a child, and remember being told, "you're too sensitive" and "don't take it personally." So I rejected certain aspects of myself and took on the role of an overachiever. I equated asking for help as a sign of weakness and decided that it was safer to do it all on my own to ensure there would never be room for someone to pull a hook, line, and sinker. I depended on no one, all the while ignoring my own need to be cared for and loved. *This is a big one for many of us, and thus the importance of Principle #8: Ask & You Shall Receive.*

He, on the other hand, took on the role of the victim. Due to false core beliefs that were instilled at an early age, it was clear that he didn't know how to communicate effectively to get his needs met properly. Somewhere in his upbringing, he hadn't learned adult life-level skills and seemed to exhibit signs of emotional immaturity; it was noticeable that he didn't handle stress well. He had a vested interest in being right all the time and used stubborn defenses over the smallest things as a way to compensate for his weak sense of self. He would frequently deflect by changing the subject—placing the blame outside himself to avoid taking responsibility and accepting accountability for his actions or lack thereof—all while failing to identify these destructive patterns and refusing to do the work.

Somewhere along the line, he had learned how to manipulate me to get the responses he needed. He talked me out of leaving a few different times, not with changed actions, not with a plan to make things better, but with hope; and I wanted so badly to believe him. When he hurt, I hurt. I found myself taking on his stuff as my own, soaking it all up like a sponge. I was loyal to a fault, even in the face of evidence that it was undeserved. Every time he gave me an excuse, I gave him the benefit of the doubt. He seemed sincere, would apologize again, then rinse and repeat—the cycle would resume. Up until this moment, I couldn't see that my compassion and kindness was being used against me.

Instead of bringing out the best of ourselves, it brought out the worst, and loving somebody unconditionally is not grounds for accepting poor behavior and blurred lines of respect. Many times, I felt smothered and bound by the words "I love you," unable to break free. I didn't need someone who claimed to love me to cause me more pain than I was already in. I refused to stay caught in the trap. I had to take responsibility, as I had allowed the toxicity. I let someone else's venom and unresolved wounds poison my spirit and my happiness. I was once again drawn into someone else's unconscious patterning and, therefore, enabled them to continue.

It's hard to see the ones we love in pain; it's only natural to want to protect them. However, we must be careful not to get too attached to their life story. When we enable someone, we hold them back from learning the lessons they need to learn, and from experiencing what they need to experience on their own journey. Only when one is forced to face the consequences of their own actions will they have the opportunity to grow. It's all about letting go of our preconceived notions and releasing the need to control the outcome—easier said than done.

The first step is to recognize you have a problem. Some of us don't give up when we are supposed to, surpassing all logic, rational, and reasoning. It seemed that the only thing sustaining the relationship was the energy I alone was putting into it—blood, sweat, and tears. I was doing myself an incredible disservice by continuing to give, over-accommodating and offering up so much of my life force, as it was hindering my healing process.

It takes two to tango; without reciprocity there is no relationship. I was tired of being put on layaway. The situation was never going to change and it was unrealistic to expect otherwise. I had to stop putting my faith in a man who wasn't ready to do the work. Time and time again, the train was leaving the station and he was choosing to not get on board. If someone's not growing with you, then they can't go with you. I realized I didn't have a choice. What I tried to hold together time and time again just fell apart. I was left with no option but to take flight, to detach from everything that didn't feel like love. I had to let go of the desire to make this relationship work, as it was a battle I could not win.

Shame on me, shame on me, for letting it go this far
Shame on me, shame on me, I took it all to heart

Take, there's no more taking to be done
Cause I have given, I have given, and got none
Still these thoughts stain the guilt on my face
I must savor what's left of me that's sane

Run, I'm running circles through my mind
See I'm leaving, yes I'm leaving this behind
Cause I've been weaving this web I call home
These scripted pages of my life are not my own

Shame on me, shame on me, for letting it go this far
Shame on me, shame on me, I took it all to heart

Hold, yes I've been holding on too tight
I'm letting go, letting go of fears I hide
Cause I am always the one to feel the pain
But in the end, I'm the only one to blame

Shame on me, shame on me, for letting it go this far
Shame on me, shame on me, I took it all to heart

And sometimes it's too late to take it back...

Shame on me, shame on me, for letting it go this far
Shame on me, shame on me, I took it all to heart

Shame on me, shame on me, for letting it go this far
Shame on me, shame on me, I took it all to heart

Shame on me, shame on me, for letting it go this far...

"Shame On Me" by Adena Sampson

Having these experiences taught me some valuable lessons that would later become the foundation for Principle #2: Surrender & Accept What Is, Principle #3: Move Through the Illusion, Principle #4: Embrace Your Vulnerability, and Principle #5: Reclaim Your Power.

The Road Back

"New beginnings are often disguised as painful endings."
— Lao Tzu

Needless to say, it didn't end well—far from the nice, neat, conscious uncoupling I would hope for from our time spent together and the soul connection we shared. The veil had been lifted—he wasn't the man he had portrayed himself to be—and I felt naïve for not recognizing it sooner. I was in a state of shock, trying to make sense of all the hurtful projections and gaslighting tactics that caused me to question the validity of our bond, our memories, and my own sanity.

For someone who seemed so strong and put together, I came apart at the seams. I had to be broken to truly surrender. It was time for this Wonder Woman to accept her own humanness and vulnerability. I had to step into the depths of my being, my core. I had to dig in and get dirty, peel away the old layers to make room for the new, like a snake shedding its skin. I was forced to lie with myself, bare naked on the floor, stripped down to the bone—die to an old way of being before being reborn.

Nature gives us such a great example of how to live. In life, there is a natural cycle of death and rebirth. The waves can be a bit bumpy and there can be some major storms. Sometimes we can get caught in a riptide, tumbled and thrown around. Most of us are looking for some smooth sailing, aren't we? We may float for a while, but it doesn't last long. Our lives are like the ocean tides, always in motion, ever changing. If we happen to be in the right place at the right time, sometimes we can catch a wave and ride it for a while. And then, it's time to catch another wave.

As we grow from our life lessons, our growth is reflected in the world around us, and many times this means new friends, new places, and a new support system. With this, however, comes a falling away—the need to let go of people, patterns, and circumstances that no longer serve us. Our sacred contract had played out and I was left finding my own closure. I needed to see the truth of the situation in order to draw a line in the sand and move forward. I can see it so clearly, now that the fog has lifted. As they say, you can't see the forest for the trees while you're in the midst of them.

I've never been one to play surface, I'm used to diving into the depths, although it is clear I can no longer allow myself to do so with people who are too scared to swim. It's taken me a while to realize that some people don't want what's best for them, but rather what's easiest for them, and wanting more for someone than they want for themselves only causes more pain. I can't help people who don't want my help, and it's not my job to fix their problems. I had to be reminded of what is mine to carry and what is not mine to carry, letting go of the old patterning of feeling the need to rescue others.

When I finally let go, I was shown the way—caught when I least expected it. I had been brought to my knees so that whatever was left unhealed could rise to the surface. All this was divinely guided, a blessing in disguise—happening *for* me, not *to* me—*which we discuss in Principle #1: Shift Your Perspective.* In the midst of being broken, I was given the gifts of fortitude, gratitude, patience, presence, and purpose. I found the strength within myself to walk by faith and not by sight, to discern fact from fiction, and to remain steadfast on the path to recovery—*which we will be discussing in greater depth in Principle #9: Have Faith Whatever It Takes.* Now I can live from a new place of understanding when all I know falls away.

It's taken an enormous amount of patience and courage to navigate all the financial, physical, emotional, psychological, and neurological effects of this disease. I feel that I've lived lifetimes within this lifetime already, and yet, I am just beginning. Through the pain, I have had many insights. I now know I have the ability within me to navigate any storm, and I am using these experiences as a huge catalyst—rising from the ashes bigger, better, and stronger than ever—ready to serve in a fuller capacity.

I am in gratitude for the love I shared with my beloveds and the dance we danced, for at the time, they were my perfect mirrors, my angels! By fully owning my shadow self, I've softened into my own humanness and now have deeper compassion and a better understanding of true surrender and a readiness to receive, reminding myself that I deserve to receive all the love and energy I give so freely into the world. I feel that I have found the fine line between unconditional love and respecting my own healthy boundaries, uncovering an ever-deeper level to loving me. I am forging ahead grateful for the lessons I've learned, excited, renewed, and connected to the flow of life and what is to come.

From nothingness comes everything. This is where creation happens. When we wipe the slate clean, we can repaint our canvas. What a great opportunity to rewrite my story, and I invite you to do the same. In the following pages, we will be discussing nine key principles: what each principle is, the benefits of each principle, how they work together to create a roadmap to help you navigate life's unexpected twists and turns, and how you can apply these principles to turn any challenge you may be facing into a victory.

I urge you to learn from your mistakes. To be open to change. To adopt the belief that everything is purposeful and happens for a reason, even if there's no tangible proof to be seen in the present moment. To practice letting go of what no longer serves you. To view rejection as a redirection, a gift, an opportunity for growth, a new beginning, making room for something bigger and better to take its place.

Keep in mind, there is no right or wrong, good or bad; it just is. For when we surrender all our judgments and perceptions, when we let go of our old programming—the old paradigms that no longer serve us—we open ourselves up to an endless array of possibilities. It's really amazing how as we grow and move forward on our journey, the roadmap seems to appear, and other aspects align and come into play. As time passes, the curtain unfolds, revealing to us our true essence and purpose in ways we never could have imagined.

PART II

THE ONLY WAY OUT IS THROUGH

"Break on through to the other side."
— THE DOORS

On the path to self-discovery, it's all about the journey. Each piece is an intricate part of the puzzle that, when put together, forms a collective whole—a masterpiece.

#1: SHIFT YOUR PERSPECTIVE

"When you change the way you look at things, the things you look at change."
— Dr. Wayne Dyer

A re you open to change? So many of us are afraid of change, but what are we so afraid of? The unknown perhaps. Change is inevitable, and it starts from within. The definition of change is to make different; cause a transformation; an event that occurs when something passes from one state to another; losing one's original nature; become different in essence.

Life is about transitions, yet many of us attempt to live in a "don't rock the boat" environment. Most of us like to feel a sense of safety and security in our lives. This sense of security is maintained by things feeling as if they are constant and unchanging. A certain amount of routine is vital for everyone; however, resistance to change is a dead-end street. If you are neither coming nor going, you are stagnant. Fear of change doesn't just hold us back, it stops us from truly living. Amidst all that is taking place in the world right now, we cannot afford to continue going down the same path. Our beliefs have created mental barriers that have caused violence, ignorance, and intolerance. Our senses are being overwhelmed and bombarded, and the repercussions are currently affecting our state of health and well-being.

When nothing is stable, the hardest thing to do is stay grounded. However, now more than ever, this is exactly what we must do. It's time to stay spiritually fit. It's time to see our life lessons in every situation, no matter how intolerable it may seem. It's time for us to take responsibility for the change we want to see in this world. It's time to think outside the box and redefine our parameters. It's time for us to come together and embrace this opportunity for growth. We can resist the change, get caught up in a whirlwind, and feel very uncomfortable, or we can learn how to cast fear aside and embrace the seasons of change. Let us use nature's wisdom to grow through life's inevitable ups and downs. It's time to tap into our inner resources, take risks, move past limitations, and be open to what lies ahead.

Rejection Is a Redirection: A Blessing in Disguise

"Looking at life from a different perspective makes you realize that it's not the deer that is crossing the road, rather it's the road that is crossing the forest."
— MUHAMMAD ALI

How many times have you found yourself in an uncomfortable circumstance, only to find out later it was a blessing in disguise?

These are ever-changing times that we live in. Now more than ever we are experiencing great shifts in energy on a global level. Right now, many of us are experiencing job losses, relationship breakups, and health issues. We are losing our homes, our loved ones, and even our own sanity. At first, it is easy to assume this is a bad thing. However, it may very well be a blessing in disguise.

Two traveling angels stopped to spend the night in the home of a wealthy family. The family was rude and refused to let the angels stay in the mansion's guest room. Instead, the angels were given a space in the cold basement. As they made their bed on the hard floor, the older angel saw a hole in the wall and repaired it. When the younger angel asked why, the older angel replied, "Things aren't always what they seem."

The next night, the pair came to rest at the house of a very poor, but very hospitable, farmer and his wife. After sharing what little food they had, the couple let the angels sleep in their bed, where they could have a good night's rest. When the sun came up the next morning, the angels found the farmer and his wife in tears. Their only cow, whose milk had been their sole income, lay dead in the field. The younger angel was infuriated and asked the older angel, "How could you have let this happen?! The first man had everything, yet you helped him," she accused. "The second family had little but was willing to share everything, and you let their cow die." "Things aren't always what they seem," the older angel replied. "When we stayed in the basement of the mansion, I noticed there was gold stored in that hole in the wall. Since the owner was so obsessed with greed and unwilling to share his good fortune, I sealed the wall so he wouldn't find it. Then last night as we slept in the farmer's bed, the angel of death came for his wife. I told him to take the cow instead. Things aren't always what they seem."

As we grow, it is reflected in the world around us, and many times this means new friends, new places, and a new support system. In these ever-shifting times, with all the ups and downs we are currently experiencing, we may find that our "old world" is no longer in alignment with the "new world" we're creating, and with this comes a falling away, the need to let go of people and circumstances that no longer serve us. The problem seems to lie in the timing of it all. It's almost as if we are dying and being reborn again while we are still alive. When we experience things ending in our life before the new has arrived, it can cause us to panic. We may feel as though all we've worked for is for naught. This can be very scary and overwhelming. Despite all our efforts, our infrastructure is falling apart, and we start to wonder how we will sustain amidst all this chaos. Which way do we go when there is no solid ground?

The first step is to adopt the belief system that everything happens for a reason. There is no such thing as a coincidence. If everything happens for a reason, then ask yourself this question: What can I learn from this, and how does this serve me?

Many of us have a tendency to allow rejection to knock us off course. We go through life continually reacting to what happens to us, always at the mercy of the ever-changing tides. Rejection is a part of life, and change the only constant; acceptance of this is key. We can't control the wind, although we can adjust our sails. We get to decide how we respond, how we navigate in any given situation. We can choose to be the victim or the victor. Just a shift in our perspective can make all the difference.

Moral of the story: *It's not happening to you, it's happening for you.* Trust that every outcome is to your advantage. Choose to see that every rejection, every so-called failed relationship, every loss, every closed door is a blessing in disguise. Remember *things aren't always what they seem*, there is more going on than meets the eye, a bigger picture with a greater purpose. Every no gets you closer to a yes. Every letdown and disappointment is leading you to something better. Life is always conspiring in our favor; we just don't always see it right away.

The Naked Truth: Reevaluating How You Measure Success

"Success is not measured by what a man accomplishes, but by the opposition he has encountered and the courage with which he has maintained the struggle against overwhelming odds."
— CHARLES LINDBERG

What is the key to success? How do we measure whether or not we are successful?

Success cannot be measured by the amount of money you make or the material assets you possess, nor from what society dictates to be the status quo. Success is what you make it; it has a certain energy about it. You can feel it in one's touch, you can hear it in one's voice, and you can see it in one's eyes.

When I got sick, I didn't have the energy to do much of anything, and yet I still had to provide for myself somehow. During that time, I didn't feel successful. Like many of us, the way I had measured success prior to losing my health, happiness, relationships, and finances was faulty. Needless to say, I ended up selling flowers while I was in Maui for cash just to get by, which at the time I knew nothing about. I quickly educated myself on the differences between orchids, plumeria, tuberose, and kukui nut leis, put a dress on, a flower behind my ear, and off I went!

I worked four nights a week and slept most of the day. I can remember a handful of people coming up to me saying, "You're my favorite flower girl, you make me smile," and the people who worked in the restaurants in Lahaina who saw me every day who said, "Your smile just makes my day!" That's when a big shift happened for me! It was in that moment that I realized the power of my presence and that true success was not measured in the way I was taught to measure success. If just my smile could make someone's day, then I was already successful doing God's work.

Looking back, my ability to pivot and do what I did was nothing short of incredible. I was being too hard on myself and judging myself by unreasonable standards. Sound familiar? We have been conditioned to seek validation through perceived success. Most of us go through life people pleasing, constantly seeking approval, whether we are aware of it or not. We have developed this pattern of pretending to be who others want us to be, just to fit in. We say to ourselves, "If I just do this, or if I just do that, then I'll be accepted." One's worth is not solely dependent on doing well, achieving things, or by doing things to please others. We must be careful not to allow outside influences to define us. So before you can achieve success, you need to define what success means to you and be willing to let go of the need to be "good enough" for everyone else.

Moral of the story: *Any shift is a big shift, so celebrate the small wins.* Don't be so hard on yourself. Remember that just a smile can make someone's day!

See the Gift in Everything: Adopting an Attitude of Gratitude

> *"Through the eyes of gratitude, everything is a miracle."*
> — MARY DAVIS

Are you ready for a miracle? When you ask for a miracle, what are you really asking for?

Most of us are asking to be shown the way. And if we are to be shown the way, then we must be open to hearing the guidance. We can't experience a miracle if we are looking for it in all the wrong places, if we are attached to the outcome and expect it to show up in a specific way or certain manner. I think many of us have this belief that a miracle is something big and majestic, something that comes out of nowhere and parts the sea only for the worthy few. That simply isn't true. Miracles are something we can experience every day.

In order for us to experience miracles more readily, we must be willing to change our mind, to think differently about the meaning we attach to our experiences. That being said, let us first define what a miracle is. One of my favorite definitions comes from *A Course in Miracles,* which states that a miracle is just a correction in perception, a decision to choose love over fear. It's merely a matter of shifting our focus.

This is a very humbling time for all of us. The current pandemic and economic crisis is a wake-up call. The good news is, what we wake up to can be greater than it was before, we just have to be willing to do our part.

I've heard so many people say that 2020 was the worst year ever. Do you agree? I'm not here to discount anyone's pain. However, it's all relative. Merely a matter of perspective. Considering I've spent the last twelve years literally fighting for my life, I can truly say that 2020 was one of the best years I've had in I can't remember when, and I don't say this lightly. Amidst all the pain and tragedy, it was a year of immense growth and transformation.

I don't say this because I was somehow more prepared, or because my circumstances were any less devastating, as I found the things around me once again falling apart. Like many of us, I lost quite a few people in my life this past year. Not to mention another business. I now know, along with countless others, what it feels like to be "nonessential."

The year 2020 affected me just as much as the next person; the only difference was, I chose to see the gifts. I chose to do the work. To look in the mirror and go within for the answers. To learn the lessons I needed to learn. To take back my power. To acknowledge my fears, gather my strength, and pivot again. The fact that I've made it this far is nothing short of a miracle. If 2020 hadn't played out as it did, I wouldn't have gotten my master's, I wouldn't have written this book. I wouldn't have gained the clarity I desperately needed to fully heal.

We have the ability to shift our perspective no matter what our circumstances and see the gift in everything. A good place to start is to adopt an attitude of gratitude. In order to create the life we want, it is important to be aware of what we already have. Some of us tend to take the simplest things for granted, like having a roof over our heads, electricity, running water, food on the table, clothes to wear, and even a car to drive. Do you realize that just by having these things you are better off than 75% of the population? Did you know that over two million people live off of less than two dollars a day? It's amazing what can happen when we focus on how blessed we truly are.

Begin each day with a grateful heart and watch the miracles unfold in your life. If you're needing a jump start, here are three powerful ways to cultivate an attitude of gratitude:

1. Visualize: Think about a time, a place, a shared emotional experience with someone that you're grateful for. Close your eyes, recall it, and really feel it...savor the moment. As you do so, you may notice a smile developing on your face. A deep sense of gratitude is known to stimulate the pleasure centers of our brains. If you practice this daily, you are cultivating more than just a quick, temporary fix; you are reprogramming your brain for a consistent, recurring experience of joy and pleasure.

2. Count Your Blessings: Make a list of everything you are grateful for. You may even want to write down the reason why you are grateful for these things. Get in the habit of going through your list before you start your day every morning. Recognize what you have and all that you have to be grateful for. Start your phrase with, "I am grateful for...." This is a powerful tool! What we focus on expands.

Gratitude is known to have lasting psychological effects on the brain, so naturally, the positive effects of feeling gratitude each day compound like interest. You may not see results immediately; however, they will gradually accrue over time, yielding a profound return on your investment.

3. Pay It Forward: Tell people how much you appreciate them. Express to others how grateful you are for their presence. It's important to show our appreciation by acknowledging the roles that other people play in our lives. Whether that's a grocery store clerk or someone who served you with extra care. Often, a simple thank you doesn't begin to truly express how you feel. Gratitude unexpressed leaves people completely unaware of the difference they've made in your life. When expressed, it leaves everyone feeling uplifted.

Research shows that there is a strong correlation between gratitude and our well-being. Gratitude can strengthen our relationships, help us accept change, and deal with adversity. It can decrease pain levels, relieve stress, reduce depression and anxiety, help us sleep better, increase energy levels, boost our happiness, and help with our overall outlook on life. By practicing gratitude daily, we're creating a powerful, positive ripple effect. We are signaling to God and the universe that we're ready to receive more miracles and abundance into our life.

Moral of the story: *Sometimes our worst moments can reveal our greatest blessings.* Cultivating an attitude of gratitude helps us see the possibilities we would have otherwise been blind to. Every day we have countless opportunities to be grateful. If we showed our gratitude for only a small portion of them, our lives would change for the better.

So the next time you find yourself lying in bed counting sheep, I invite you to count your blessings instead. Take time to reflect. Be curious. How are you currently living your day-to-day life? Are you part of the solution? Or part of the problem? What are you grateful for? What can you do to appreciate the things you already have in your life?

Don't forget that every morning when you wake up, you have a choice. You can get up and say, "Oh God, it's another day" or you can say, "Thank you, God, for another day!" Choose to shift your perspective, reframe your experiences, change the way you look at things so that the things you look at change. Live life to its fullest in deep gratitude. Make every moment and every second count. Choose to see the miracle, the gift in everything.

To sum up this first principle, I leave you with an excerpt from the *Daily Word*: "I no longer try to change outer things. They are simply a reflection. I change my inner perception and the outer reveals the beauty so long obscured by my own attitude. I concentrate on my inner vison and find my outer view transformed. I find myself attuned to the grandeur of life and in unison with the perfect order of the universe."

#2 SURRENDER & ACCEPT WHAT IS

"Surrender isn't about giving up or giving in; it's about giving over."

— JUDITH ORLOFF

H ave you ever noticed that when you cling too tightly to something, someone, or a situation, it eludes you? So why do we try to control the outcome? Why do we make life harder than it really needs to be? We've all heard the saying "what we resist, persists," so why do we continue to push down doors when we can walk through the open ones?

Many things happen in our lives that are outside of our control. When they do, we have two choices: We can choose to fight against it and try to change it, or surrender to it and accept what is. Unfortunately, most of us were taught to believe that surrendering means defeat. The word *surrender* tends to have negative connotations associated with it due to its use in the context of war. Surrendering does not mean that you've lost the battle, actually quite the contrary. It is not a sign of weakness; it is a pillar of strength. It means letting go of certain behaviors, people, and circumstances that no longer serve you. It means surrendering to the war in your mind so that you may be at peace.

Surrendering is all about letting go of our preconceived notions and releasing the need to control the outcome. There's a difference between needing to know the way and allowing yourself to be shown the way. In order for grace to enter our lives, we must make room for forces beyond our control. We must let go of our desire to control the outcome and surrender to it. The truth is control is an illusion, and when we try to maintain control, we suffer.

Surrendering is about being present, living moment to moment in the flow. What do I mean by flow? It's a simple concept really. The Taoists, for example, believe that God is within us and all around us, in everyone and everything. We are all energy and energy is always in motion, in flux, in flow. For so long now, many of us have lived like salmon swimming upstream. Wouldn't it be easier to just go in the direction of the current, the flow? What stops us from going with the flow? I'll give you one guess…it's fear. When we are in fear, even if just a moment, we are disconnected from source. When we surrender, we are swimming in the Tao, dancing with the universe.

The way the universe works is far more simple than most imagine. We first have to know exactly what we want, ask for it, then detach from it completely. The universe does the rest. It's really as simple as that. When we are putting too much effort forth, there is no room for God to step in and help. We have to take action and put forth the effort. However, not to the point where we're so attached to the outcome that we override what's in our highest good. Many of us come from a mindset of scarcity. When we have an underlying belief that things in life don't come easily; we tend to hold on too tightly and fight harder for those things. When we fight against the current, we push away the very thing that we say we want. When we surrender to it, we send out a signal that says we are ready to receive.

Surrendering gives us a chance to stand back and view situations in life with greater clarity. We can't control the variables, but we can control our response to them. It comes down to trusting in yourself and your abilities and having faith that it will all work out.

So I invite you to let go and let God. Stop trying so hard to control things. Instead of struggling against nature, accept it and work with it. Detach from the outcome completely and let life work its magic. Make room for miracles. Release any doubt, fear, or worry that is attached to having the things that you desire. Know you're why, put it out there, then leave room for how it's delivered.

Rome Wasn't Built in a Day: A Little Patience Can Go a Long Way

"To be at peace in any endeavor, we must release our need to control the outcome."
— DIANE DREHER

They say patience is a virtue. I sure wasn't born with it, were you?

What does it mean to have patience? Patience is defined as the capacity to accept or tolerate delay, trouble, or suffering without getting angry or upset. It's the ability to wait. To continue doing something despite difficulties. To bear annoyance without complaint. Patience involves perseverance and requires a certain level of endurance.

We, as a whole, have become a society based on agendas and instant gratification. Seems like we are always on the run and in such a hurry to get things done. As an overachiever, I know the feeling all too well of wanting to go straight from point A to point Z without having to take all the steps along the way, all the while second-guessing myself, thinking I'm running behind, and wondering how I can get further along. The impatience we feel often occurs in response to some sort of delay in life that is not going according to our expectation. For example, getting stuck in traffic or waiting on someone who's running late. Life can't be lived without encountering something that interferes with our plans, so it's helpful when we can learn to surrender to and accept these disruptions as a normal part of life rather than expecting otherwise.

This reminds me of the time when I sold everything I owned and packed up and moved to Maui. In order to bring over as many items of clothing that I could, I did what most women would never dream of: I rolled my clothes. Yes, all of them. Including this two-piece red suit that I was planning on wearing for a business presentation I was giving at the Maui Arts & Cultural Center in two days. Upon arrival, one of the first things I did was head to the local dry cleaners. I got up to the counter to explain why I needed this specific item dry-cleaned and said, "Can you rush this please?" They looked at me like I was from outer space. "I'm sorry, ma'am, we have to send that out to Lahaina and that takes about four days."

When I left the dry cleaners, I started to laugh at myself. Coming from Las Vegas, I hadn't realized how blessed I was to be able to drive through the dry cleaners. I was used to pulling up at the drive-through window, tipping them a few extra bucks, and going about my day. I share this story because it was another pivotal moment that really allowed me to see things more clearly. Just when I thought I was going with the flow, I get to the dry cleaners only to be blatantly reminded that I still had quite a ways to go.

Moral of the story: *Life's a journey, not a destination. A marathon, not a sprint.* So enjoy the ride. Be patient. Take it step-by-step. Remember, every step in between is pertinent to our growth. Every step of the way, we learn something new. If we skip a step, we may miss an amazing opportunity that we fail to notice, because we are in such a hurry to climb.

The Power of Acceptance: Managing Expectations

"Acceptance is the answer to all my problems today. When I am disturbed, it is because I find some person, place, thing, or situation—some fact of my life—unacceptable to me, and I can find no serenity until I accept that person, place, thing, or situation as being exactly the way it is supposed to be at this moment. Nothing, absolutely nothing happens in God's world by mistake. Unless I accept life completely on life's terms, I cannot be happy. I

need to concentrate not so much on what needs to be changed in the world as on what needs to be changed in me and in my attitudes."
— *THE BIG BOOK*

Do you ever catch yourself saying, "I should" do this or "I should" do that? Do you often feel let down?

Holding onto the preconceived notions of how things "should" be doesn't serve. Most of us make decisions based on what we believe we should do rather than what we want to do. Expectations have been heavily ingrained in our society and we learn to adopt them very early on in life. Expectations quite often can cause problems, for when they are not met we become disappointed, and all too often, they are never met. This is how we set ourselves up for failure. Our egos get so hung up on expecting people to act and behave a certain way, and when they don't we throw a pity party.

Most of us don't even realize that we are projecting our reality onto others. All too often, we can have unreasonable expectations of ourselves that are unhealthy. We can be our own worst critic and therefore it can be hard to escape our own attitudes, for they form the nature of what we see. Many of us developed a need for control early on in life as a coping mechanism for the fear of the unknown, a way of compensating for the instability and uncertainty we felt at home. We are convinced that some part of our life should be some other way than it is, and that the people in it should be some other way than they are.

Since I can remember, I've always had great expectations of myself and others. I've always been a stickler about showing up ahead of time or at the very least on time to any sort of meeting. Prior to honing in on patience as a virtue, I had adopted the belief early on in life that if I wanted something done I would have to do it myself, otherwise it wouldn't get done, or at least not up to my standards.

The day of the big presentation came and I remember looking at the clock wondering where everyone was, as I knew we had gotten the word out in plenty of time. My good friend Rodney Allgood, who had invited me to share the stage with him, was one of the top leaders in the company we were both involved with at the time. He assured me that we would have a packed house and that everyone was just on Hawaiian time, having a relaxed attitude towards matters of punctuality.

This was no joke. First the wardrobe malfunction, and now this. As I recall, we didn't start the meeting until about a half an hour later than we were supposed to start. You can imagine at the time how painful this was for me, as I was taught anyone who showed up late wasn't allowed in. Once again, I had no choice but to hang loose, be flexible, and surrender my expectations of the way I thought things "should" be. If I hadn't been adaptable and gone with the flow, we wouldn't have had such a successful event.

It's in times like these where we must practice the art of allowing, surrendering to, and accepting what is. Here are a few tips to help you with this process:

- Identify Where You Need to Surrender: Are you focused on the things that you can directly influence? Or are you too busy focusing on someone else's business? The reason why we try to control things is because of what we think will happen if we don't. Control is rooted in fear. Therefore, it's important to pinpoint the fear and question its validity. What are you afraid will happen if you let go of control?

- Loosen Your Grip: If you're still holding on, you may have overstayed your welcome. Change is a constant, and control is only an illusion. The need to control stems from being attached to a specific outcome, and although at times we may have influence in certain situations, we have absolutely no control over them. The only thing we do have control over is how we respond. Therefore, our attempts to control people and situations is exactly what causes our suffering. When we stop depending on others so that we can feel good, we set ourselves free.

- Live in the Moment: Love is acceptance for what is, right now, in the present moment. Some of us make the mistake of living in the future, looking forward to all our expectations. When we do so, we overlook the treasures of today. We must allow people and situations to be just as they are, without wanting to fix them or change them. When we let go of our expectations for a particular outcome, we open ourselves up to an array of endless possibilities as we learn to appreciate the true beauty of the moment, the true beauty in others, and the true beauty within ourselves.

Moral of the story: *Don't "should" on yourself or others, it's messy.* Remember you have a choice. You "could" do this or you "could" do that. So reclaim your power! Practice seeing things in a different light. Let go of what doesn't serve you and make space for something new to emerge. Take personal responsibility to create the future you envision, above and beyond expectations.

Life's a Dance: Destiny Vs. Choice

"The journey between what you once were and who you are now becoming is where the dance of life really takes place."
— BARBARA DE ANGELIS

Do you have any regrets? Have you ever thought that if you had gone left instead of going right things would be different?

Maybe you could have fixed this, could have stopped that. When we do this to ourselves, this is where the pain comes in. When we revisit the past, we can experience feelings of guilt, and feeling fear always comes from worrying about the future. Hence the value of the present moment, for when we are living in the present moment we are dancing with the universe.

Let's bring up the subject of destiny versus choice. In life, is it destiny that decides our fate or our free will? If you believe it's choice, then you regard your life as a product of your own decisions. If you believe in destiny, you believe that there are greater forces defining your life story. Why does it have to be one or the other? What if it's both?

It is here that I am reminded of a dear friend of mine who often says, "Yes and…" when deciding on what fun we will be getting into. His lighthearted reflection is a perfect reminder that it doesn't have to be one way or the other. It takes two to tango. A partnership. Dancing requires balance, grace, movement, anticipation, surrender. I believe life is a combination of both destiny and choice coexisting together as one.

Think of it this way: Destiny is a roadmap created by the universe that shows you where your life can lead. Our free will gives us choices regarding that roadmap. You may choose to take the road less traveled by—the scenic route rather than the interstate. Just know that wherever you are on your journey, all roads lead the way home.

So the next time you're second-guessing yourself, I invite you to dance. Take the stage and do your part. Put on some music and feel the beat. Dance to the rhythm of your own heart and let it lead the way. Remind yourself that growth isn't always linear. Sometimes you take two steps forward and one step back. Irrelevant, each step you take serves a purpose. There are no mistakes, no coincidences. So trust all is as it should be.

In the words of country music artist John Michael Montgomery, "Life's a dance you learn as you go, sometimes you lead sometimes you follow." It's how we choose to move with it that makes all the difference!

#3: MOVE THROUGH THE ILLUSION

"To be beautiful means to be yourself. You don't need to be accepted by others. You need to accept yourself."
— THICH NHAT HANH

W hat is beauty? What defines what we deem to be beautiful? Beauty is in the eye of the beholder. This statement shows us that our perception plays a big role in how we view life and what we may consider beautiful. How we perceive things has to do with our beliefs. Most of us develop our beliefs based on what we were taught at a young age. We tend to carry those beliefs and preconceived ideas with us, whether or not they are true. The extent of our knowledge creates our reality because the mind can only contemplate that which it has been exposed to, hence the illusion.

Sometimes our mind is our greatest enemy. This is the opposite of what most people would think—"think" being the key word here. You know that little voice in your head that keeps popping up? I know, now you're thinking which one, right? The one that's always criticizing you, reinforcing the false belief that you're "not good enough." The one that's playing small, self-doubting you saying, "You can't do this." The one that downplays your achievements saying, "It's no big deal." Ego's voice always has a way of putting up a fight. Overanalyzing and overthinking something can lead us into distress, or put us in a mild state of schizophrenia thinking we have truly lost our minds. Which brings me to a point... in order to be at peace, isn't that what we must do? Lose our minds.

Many times, our negative self-talk is the main cause of our anxiety, depression, and anger. Our inner critic evolved over the years through various forms of faulty programming as a coping strategy in response to our childhood experiences. It was initially formed to help us avoid rejection, pain, and shame—to win approval from our parents. Hence why some of these automatic narratives continue to replay in our minds as adults and can be a hard habit to break. Unfortunately, we are so used to negative feedback that we are more aware of our weaknesses than our strengths.

How we see ourselves can have a big impact on our self-esteem, and our self-esteem reflects our overall worth. Our inner critic can appear to reflect the truth, which makes it convincing. It tries to convince us that we are not worthy of love. Our inner critic can have us believe that we're not deserving of love and that we are better off on our own. This simply isn't true, for these critical thoughts are not based in reality.

Oftentimes, our inner critic is at its loudest when we are navigating uncharted territory, so it's important to learn how to discern fact from fiction and find our own truth. To differentiate between our perception and reality. To free ourselves from the bias of negativity and anything else that is blocking our clear vison.

Changing our relationship with our inner critic is a process. It doesn't happen overnight. However, the sooner we take steps towards freeing ourselves from our inner critic, the sooner we will experience the confidence and success we deserve.

1. Notice Your Inner Critic: Become aware of your internal dialogue—how you speak to yourself. When something doesn't go well—say you dropped something or made a mistake—what's your knee-jerk immediate reaction? Notice any over-the-top harsh phrases. For instance, perhaps you catch yourself saying things like "that was stupid" or "shame on you!" It's also important to take note of how you may dismiss, minimize, and downplay your accomplishments.

2. Free Your Mind: We are more powerful than we give ourselves credit for. We must take responsibility for what we are thinking, for what we are thinking creates how we are feeling. When we learn to shift our perspective about the things we think are problems, everything changes. So try giving your inner critic a name. Choose something funny, something silly, something off-putting that lacks credibility. For instance, you could name it after a

character from one of your favorite TV shows, movies, or novels. Perhaps you go with Gollum from *The Lord of the Rings* or Ethel from the classic *I Love Lucy* episodes. Either way, naming our inner critic helps us separate from our negative thought patterns. When we identify our inner critic as something outside of ourselves by approaching our thinking with a lighthearted mindset, we take away its power instead of buying into its critical dialogue as undisputable truth.

3. Practice Self-Compassion: Don't be so hard on yourself. Recognize that you're a work in progress. Remind yourself that you're ever evolving. Acknowledge your inner critic, thank it for sharing, and then stand up to it. Practice self-regulating without judgment. Replace judgment with curiosity. Speak kindly to yourself. Treat yourself with the same care, generosity, and loving-kindness as you would a dear friend. Respond instead with "It's okay, don't worry about it" or "It's no big deal, it's not the end of the world." Research suggests that practicing self-compassion is linked to a greater sense of self-worth. Also, when we practice the art of self-compassion, we are more likely to bounce back quicker after a setback.

4. Be Your Own Cheerleader: Stop waiting for other people's approval to acknowledge your victories. Give yourself credit where credit is due. Many times we can get so caught up in reaching the end goal that we forget to acknowledge the little steps and achievements along

the way. So take time to celebrate how far you've come before continuing on to your next goal. Give yourself a pep talk and pat yourself on the back for a job well done.

So I invite you to catch yourself the next time your inner critic speaks. Notice what thoughts and emotions come up. Aspire to seek the truth. Question your beliefs and preconceived notions. Practice guiding your thoughts towards loving yourself. Change how you treat yourself. Choose to think, speak, and act on purpose. Remember, you can create an inner landscape that is a match to how you want to feel. Just free your mind and the rest will follow.

Lifting the Veil: Overcoming Self-Sabotage

"Your task is not to seek for love, but merely to seek and find all the barriers within yourself that you have built against it."
— RUMI

Do you believe that you are worthy of love? Do you use your past as an excuse for your current behavior?

Our subconscious mind has a lot of evidence from our past experiences to hold us hostage. If we have an underlying subconscious belief that we're not worthy, our mind will go to great lengths to prove to us that we are right. Our ego thinks it's protecting us from danger, although it's really just keeping us from being happy. In an attempt to protect ourselves, we engage in destructive impulsive behavior that doesn't serve us. This self-sabotage is misguided love and often occurs in situations that involve a great deal of commitment. It often rises to the surface in unseen and unpredictable ways, keeping us from having fulfilling relationships and achieving our goals.

How do you know if you're sabotaging yourself? If you're not moving in the direction of what it is you say you want, you are most likely engaging in self-sabotaging behavior. When we engage in self-sabotaging behavior, there's an underlying conflict in our personality, a disconnect between our will and our actions. It is the act of preventing yourself from succeeding at what you're trying to accomplish.

The first step to overcoming self-sabotaging behavior is to identify it. Self-sabotaging behavior is not always easy to spot and can show up in a myriad of ways:

- Self-betrayal

- Pushing people away

- Isolating when you're in pain

- Refusing to ask for help

- Underestimating your worth

- Unable to receive compliments

- Comparing yourself to others

- Obsessing over the negative

- Playing the blame game

- Picking fights

- Dating people who aren't right for you

- Continually putting other people's needs before your own

- Using excuses to procrastinate

- Allowing fear to keep you stuck

- Numbing through addiction

- Running away when things don't go smoothly

When these self-sabotaging behavioral patterns repeat, which unfortunately at first they will, we have a choice. We can move forward and make a conscious decision to choose differently next time and each time the opportunity comes around to test us, or we can choose to stay stuck, since this requires no work, and choose the easy way out by running away. At some point in our lives, choosing to ignore what keeps coming up is only going to cause us more pain by recreating time and again what is inevitably unhealthy. The outcome solely depends on choice.

The key to having a good relationship starts from within. We must remove our old programming, clearing out any deep-rooted, outdated beliefs that are blocking us from experiencing real love. We need to shift our perspective about past experiences and learn to regulate self-sabotaging behaviors. In order to do this, we must take responsibility for our own emotions and reactions instead of placing the blame outside ourselves. To blame each other only keeps us in pain and allows us to avoid the real truth. In running away from our truth, we create the opposite of what we truly want.

It takes courage to face our own dysfunction and do away with self-sabotaging behavior. It requires us to reflect, get intimate with our fears, and take responsibility for our actions or the lack thereof. Being able to participate in unconditional love stems from how much we are willing to love ourselves. It's about owning our worth and honoring ourselves fully, being careful not to sacrifice our emotional needs in order to keep the peace.

So the next time you catch yourself involved in some sort of self-sabotaging behavior, I invite you to take some time to reflect and adjust your approach. Ask yourself if this behavior is truly supporting you. Take note of any fearful narratives that might be playing out behind the scenes. By taking your own inventory, you will start to see yourself with greater clarity. Remember to be compassionate during this process. You're only holding yourself back by beating yourself up. Practice being self-loving instead of self-sacrificing. Let go of any past wounds that no longer serve you, and be open to becoming the love that you so much desire.

Identifying Your Fearful Narratives: Rewriting Your Story

"Loving ourselves through the process of owning our story is the bravest thing we'll ever do."
— BRENE BROWN

What's your story? What are you choosing as your reality?

There is an ancient mantra that says, "the truth shall set you free," and the truth is the world is nothing but our perception of it. This imagined truth creates our distorted reality. We see and hear only through the filter of our past data, our story. Our story is what we tell ourselves over and over again. We use it to justify our actions and we continue to tell the same story again and again to anyone who will listen. We hang on to what's familiar because we feel it keeps us safe, but it really causes us to suffer. Our pain comes from clinging too tightly to what we've been taught and told. In order to experience true freedom, we must uncover the lies we've been telling ourselves about who we are.

In order to move through the illusion and see clearly, we must be willing to acknowledge our story and then let it go completely, and that's difficult because when this happens we feel like everything is falling apart. When everything falls apart, we can be left in an uncomfortable place where fear resides, desperately grasping for something familiar and solid to hold onto. Often in this space we lack confidence, feel stuck, and are unsure of how to move forward.

One of the main reasons many of us get stuck and are unable to move forward is due to our fear of the unknown, which brings up feelings of uncertainty. Some of our fears are healthy and rational in nature, say when our physical safety is threatened. For example, having a fear of heights prevents us from getting too close to the edge of a cliff or architectural structure. These kinds of fears are an adaptive response to help us survive, to keep us safe, and to be alert to danger.

However, there are some fears that have no rhyme or reason and only arise when our ego is threatened. These types of fears can be more subtle and less tangible in nature. They can motivate us into action or stop us dead in our tracks. An example of this is having a fear of success or a fear of failure. Rarely do these self-generated fears stem from the truth.

Our thoughts can be our worst instigator, as our conditioned mind has a way of playing tricks on us by feeding us false evidence that appears real. When we project into the future, we experience a reality that doesn't exist. For example, a fear that your partner is having an affair. Your partner may very well be cheating on you. However, this is not always the case and can very well be a reflection of the way you feel about yourself. These types of false assumptions can lead us to feeling hopeless and anxious. Life is hard enough without adding our fearful narratives into it.

Whether our narratives work for us or against us depends solely on the limiting beliefs, doubts, and fears that are playing out in our subconscious mind. Our unacknowledged fears can cause a lot of damage, so it is important that we become aware of them. When we are able to acknowledge our fears and bring them to the surface, we are then able to override them by reframing them and interpreting them from a higher perspective. That being said, here is a simple yet powerful five-step process to help you do just that.

1. Center Yourself: Make sure you're in a quiet space. Grab a pen and paper and then take a slow deep breath in and out.

2. Identify Your Fearful Narratives & Limiting Beliefs: What are the limiting beliefs that are keeping you in a state of fear? What fearful narratives have been running beneath the surface for years affecting all areas of your life? Take a moment to write down anything that come to mind. This should be done swiftly, without thinking

too much or trying too hard, in order for it to flow freely from your subconscious mind. For example: "I'm not good enough," "No one understands me," "I'm scared of moving forward," "I am afraid to rock the boat."

3. Dig a Little Deeper: Take each fear, each limiting belief and ask yourself why you believe this, why you are afraid, then write down your reasoning. For example, "I am afraid that if I move forward (work on myself, love myself, change), I will lose relationships with those I care for."

4. Explore the Origin: For each item on your list, think about these questions: What is your earliest memory of this? What event may have triggered it? In what circumstances do you find yourself anxious and uneasy? In what ways has having this fear and/or limiting belief affected your life? List both positive and negative aspects.

5. Reframe & Affirm: Challenge your preexisting thinking. Take this list and acknowledge your fears while realizing it is not the truth. Do this by taking your pen and running a single line through your limiting beliefs. Then, on a separate sheet of paper, write the exact opposite down. For example, "I am good enough," "I am full of confidence," "I am the best communicator," "I am fully understood." Post these affirmative statements on sticky notes on your mirror or refrigerator, on a whiteboard or on your wall, or just lay it by your bedside so that you can

access what you have written. Read these affirmations aloud daily, first thing upon rising and right before you go to bed at night. These are the best times to access and reprogram the subconscious mind.

When we shift our perspective, our fearful narratives no longer have control over us. So the next time you find yourself paralyzed by fear, ask yourself: Is this fear mine? Is it rational? Is it true? How can I change my relationship with this fear? Reflecting on our fears can help us discover their origins, their purpose, and why we hold onto them. This process can help us appreciate the ways our fears have kept us safe while also giving us an opportunity to reframe them. We have to change our point of view in order to change our limiting beliefs.

Mastering Uncertainty: Tapping into the Courage That Lies Within

"It's not the problem that causes our suffering; it's our thinking about the problem."
— BYRON KATIE

When all your hands have been dealt and all your chips are down, what do you do? Do you feel weak, smaller somehow, somewhat less than?

Many of us want to embody confidence before we are willing to go through the process of what it takes to actually get there. Confidence improves with competence. The more you do something, the better you become. Confidence breeds confidence; it comes from experience, and every step is cumulative. In order to fuel our self-confidence, we must first take action to prove we can feel confident in taking the next step. In essence, confidence is a decision we make to master uncertainty, to build our self-belief.

That being said, here are a few tips to help you build your self-belief, gain more confidence, and master uncertainty:

- Adopt a Beginner's Mindset: When we start doing something that we've never done before, we're starting at the very beginning of our journey, and we often get ourselves into trouble when we compare ourselves to those who are ahead of us on the journey. When we are looking into the future we are not present, and when we are not present we can find ourselves feeling overwhelmed with what may seem like insurmountable obstacles. We judge ourselves as if there is something wrong with where we are currently at on our journey. That's when self-doubt creeps in, and more often than not, procrastination is to follow. So stop comparing your chapter one to someone else's chapter twenty. Cut yourself some slack. You don't learn to ride a bike without trial and error. More often than not, you falter—you fall down and scrape your knee a few times before you feel confident enough in your bike-riding abilities—and then, before you know it, you're having the time of your life standing up and zipping down that hill!

- Do What Scares You: You must be willing to face your fears head-on and take imperfect, courageous action, for doing so will help you gain the necessary skills and confidence to deal with it more effectively. So start by making a list of a few things that scare you. Then stretch yourself by committing to taking action on those fears. Start small. For instance, if you're afraid of having an uncomfortable conversation with someone to address an issue, have the conversation. If you're uncomfortable say, going out to eat on your own, schedule a date with yourself once a week and slowly let this experience build your self-confidence. Anytime we step outside our comfort zone, we grow from our courage.

• Get Comfortable with the Uncomfortable: In order to master our feelings of uncertainty and propel ourselves forward, we must increase our tolerance to our discomfort by leaning into it, not running away from it. We need to know that an uncomfortable feeling is not the enemy. It's a gift that says, "get honest; inquire." So instead of resisting it—which only gives you short-term relief—practice focusing on how you can grow and benefit from it. When you allow life's inevitable uncomfortable moments to be part of your learning process, you're teaching yourself to handle whatever life throws your way.

• Don't Be Afraid to Make Mistakes: Because there are no mistakes. Everything happens for a reason, so don't let your "perceived" mistakes intimidate you. Sometimes it helps to gain some perspective; what's the worst that can happen? If you don't try, you'll never succeed and you'll never know unless you try. In order to bridge the gap between our perception and reality, we must be willing to take risks, try new things, and venture into the unknown…allowing ourselves to navigate and course-correct along the way.

While on this journey called life, sometimes we can get off track. We take winding roads that lead us astray, and this can make us feel like we've lost our way. We find ourselves calling out, reaching for something or someone to lend us a hand and guide us back home. It is in those moments that we can rest assured that even the detours are in divine order and for our highest good. Remember everything happens for a reason. It all comes down to trusting in yourself and your abilities, having faith that it will all work out. In this place of uncertainty lies the opportunity to be reborn and start new, for it's in this void and out of this nothingness that we can create anything we desire.

So I invite you to look into the truth of the matter. Dig in deep and end the game, the charade, the façade. Wipe the slate clean, let it all go, let it all fall apart, let it all wash away and then rewrite your story. Be brave. Step out of who you thought you were and into who you are meant to be. Life is about taking risks. We learn from our experiences, so get out there and experience. Have the courage to leap and take the plunge, spread your wings and fly. For sometimes what you're most afraid of doing is the very thing that will set you FREE!

As the late Mark Twain once said, "Courage is not the absence of fear. It is acting in spite of it."

#4: EMBRACE YOUR VULNERABILITY

"The imperfections of a man, his frailties, his faults, are just as important as his virtues. You can't separate them. They're wedded."
— HENRY MILLER

Are you a perfectionist? Do you try to cover up your perfection in an attempt to appear perfect? Many of us have days when we know we aren't at our best. Maybe we're feeling tired and overwhelmed. In those moments, do you catch yourself apologizing for your behavior as if the way you are "being" is unacceptable, not good enough in some way?

As human beings, we seem to place conditions on our love. We know not what we do. Once again, a lot of this stems from our childhood from what we were taught was socially acceptable or unacceptable. The true meaning of unconditional love is love given without conditions. So in order to love unconditionally, we need to set aside the conditions that we put on our love. For example, letting go of the need for other people to act or behave in a certain way. As perfectionists, we expect those around us to be perfect, and we already know that doesn't work. Instead, why not work on accepting others just the way they are, imperfectly perfect.

In order to do this, you must first accept yourself, flaws and all. This means recognizing the part that you play in any given situation. It means owning up to your mistakes without beating yourself up. It means having no regrets, releasing all shame and all guilt. It means showing up as your authentic self, acknowledging your shortcomings, and celebrating your strengths.

What would your life be like if you appreciated your imperfections as the very essence of your being, as your signature makeup? Stop and think for a moment of something that you just adore. For example, your favorite shirt that has a hole in it, or your favorite ceramic piece that has a crack on the side. These certain qualities are exactly what gives it character and meaning. The colors, the textures, the richness. So why would you want to replace it with something else? The same goes for you. You are unique. Your scars tell a story. Your soul has its own frequency, and there's nothing more beautiful than simply being your true authentic self.

Authenticity is rare, and it is time for that to change. The masks we wear prevent us from creating the life we want, from reaching our goals and unlocking our true potential. Radical authenticity begins from within, with the ability to remain present, being able to go into any moment without role play. In order to do this, we must get raw and real and embrace our vulnerability, delve deep within the spaces of resistance and swim into the unknown, naked but unembarrassed.

Unfortunately, we live in a culture that tends to view vulnerability as weakness and are often criticized for it. We've been conditioned to believe that specific facets of ourselves are unacceptable. There's a battle going on inside us, between who we are being and who we want to be. We tend to see things in black or white, right or wrong, good or bad without making room for the variances in between. It's an ego struggle and it comes down to lack of self-acceptance. This narrow-minded, self-righteous judgment needs to stop! We must stop measuring ourselves by unreasonable standards. We cannot be afraid to look in the mirror and admit to ourselves our frailties. For without the darkness, we wouldn't be able to recognize the light.

It's time for us as a collective to lose our minds and get reacquainted with our hearts. It's time for us to embrace our vulnerability, making room for a larger view, a broader spectrum, for both the light and dark within us. Embracing our vulnerability is the most powerful thing we can do. When we get deeply familiar with our pain, making peace with our shadow without judgment, it gives other people permission to do the same.

So I invite you to uncover your authentic self. Lift up your mask, take off your cape, and lay down your shield. For even Wonder Woman and Superman need a break. Stop seeking outside yourself for approval and validation, let go of all judgments, and allow yourself to just be.

Be Honest

Keep the parts of your identity that serve you and shed the parts that don't. For example, your adaptive self may have a pattern of telling little white lies, whether out of convenience, to further an agenda, or to save face. Our culture seems to have the false belief that telling a white lie does no harm, that it's somehow no big deal. It's imperative we stop justifying dishonesty and maintain alignment between what we say and what we do. Telling any type of lie robs us and those we love of our authentic selves. When we mask our true identities, our true intentions, we not only violate someone else's trust, we also bruise our character.

Remember, the more lies we tell, the less accepting we are of our authentic self. So commit to your evolution. Ask yourself why you feel the need to lie. Perhaps you're afraid of hurting someone, or you're afraid of being rejected. We all want to be liked, but at what cost? Is it worth losing your self-respect?

Being honest with others starts with being honest with ourselves. It requires that we allow ourselves to be seen in all our imperfect messiness. So practice letting go of the lies that are holding you back and get in the habit of telling the truth. Start small. For instance, the next time a stranger asks how you are doing, see if you can override your habitual response of "I'm great, thank you, and you?" to whatever is true for you in that moment. For example, say you just found out that your friend has died. An honest response may sound like, "I'm having a rough day, just lost a dear friend of mine." By being honest and admitting our frailties, we create closeness and connection with others, and peace and confidence within ourselves.

Be True

Are you being who you want to be? Authentic individuals are considered trustworthy because they do what they say they are going to do, they walk the walk. So it's important to take the time to explore what your core values are (what you consider important in life) and ask yourself if your actions are correctly reflecting them.

Perhaps you value adventure, community, family, freedom. Maybe it's honesty, justice, kindness, knowledge. It could be leadership, love, loyalty, peace, pleasure, recognition, security, spirituality. Whatever your values, it's important to identify any external situations that may trigger you to veer away from them.

For example, let's say you value kindness although you often find yourself saying mean things to your partner anytime you get in a heated argument. It might behoove you to be aware of the excuses you use to justify this behavior and take note of any discrepancies between your actions and your beliefs. Ask yourself why these situations lead you astray. Oftentimes it's because there's a conflict between living our values and getting our needs met.

For instance, you may have adopted this defensive coping mechanism earlier on in life in an attempt to keep you feeling safe. So take a moment to reflect on what needs are being met when you go against your core values. How else could you get these needs met? Once we identify our values and acknowledge any gaps in between living them and getting our needs met, we can then practice making decisions that are more in alignment, bridging the gap and paving the way towards the authentic person that we want to be.

Be You

Be open and vulnerable enough to lay it all on the line. Risk being seen, get naked, put yourself out there, let loose. Recognize that developing authenticity and self-acceptance takes time. There is no shortcut; it's a daily practice, an ongoing process. So do something bold, something silly, something imperfectly perfect each and every day to uncover, own, unleash, and nurture your authentic self.

Practice stating your opinions and accepting your preferences. For instance, if you are being asked where you would like to go eat, instead of being indifferent try stating what you would prefer. Practice acknowledging your needs. Perhaps you just need a hug, so muster up the courage and ask for one. Practice accepting your emotions. Transformation doesn't come from a place of denial; it comes from a place of acceptance. So shine a light into the darkness. Observe what comes up for you without judgment.

For example, you may have said things and done things during times of intense pain, anxiety, and depression that upon reflection you were horrified by. You may have even scared yourself, wondering if these outbursts revealed a much darker, sinister side of your persona, a side that is not seen when in better health. It may have left you feeling regretful, guilty, and ashamed. It's important when this happens to practice witnessing these feelings objectively. We all experience negative emotions;

we wouldn't be human if we didn't. So treat yourself like a caring, compassionate friend would. Be leery of any spiritual and religious dogmas that seek to condemn or deny what it means to be human.

Remember what we resist, persists. The more we avoid our darkness, the more it grows within us, and the more fragmented we become. Instead of denying its existence, it's important we explore the dark, hidden crevices within our psyche and take ownership of them, for the repression of our shadow self is one of the biggest barriers towards authenticity and self-love. When we learn to integrate and embrace these disconnected parts of ourselves, we become whole and better equipped to handle adversity. So make peace with your shadow self and accept your own humanness: the good, the bad, and the ugly at its core. Love all aspects of you, because until you do, no one else will. The more you stop trying to be perfect, the more you will discover just how perfect you really are.

Unlocking Your True Potential: Celebrating Your Greatness

"You reclaim your power by loving what you were once taught to hate."
— BRYANT H. McGILL

What is your superpower? Hint: It's not a skill, it's a perspective. It's often something that really bothers you, something unjust that you're willing to take a stand for, something that motivates you to rise up against it. It's not what you do or what you say, it's just who you are. A way of being that enhances everything you touch. Your particular genius. Your secret sauce. Something that people look to you for.

Many times it's hard to see our superpowers (our strengths, the gifts that make us truly special), as they are often covered up by our insecurities (our inner nemesis). Sadly, we have a tendency to focus far too much on the negative aspects of our special abilities and may even consider them to be a weakness (a curse). This is our kryptonite! It could very well be the one thing you were criticized for growing up. The one thing that wasn't viewed as a compliment. The one thing you may have put on the list of things that you thought were inherently wrong with you. Often the gifts we wind up contributing to the world have to do with a time of pain we've lived through. At first, our superpowers may feel like a heavy burden to bear, especially when we're not fully aware of and aligned with the gifts that they bring.

When I was younger, I was told that I was too sensitive, too intense because I felt things so deeply. My sensitivity was my vulnerability. Oftentimes I placed other people's needs before my own. I cared "too much" and people who sensed my weak boundaries used my innate kindness as a means to their end. In my romantic relationships, I never felt I had enough space. I often felt smothered and stifled as it wasn't easy separating my feelings from the feelings of others.

If you are a highly sensitive person like myself, life has probably felt hard, disheartening, and painful at times because you feel so deeply. You may have even tried to disown your sensitivity because you just can't see how to sustain your light in such a heavy world. You may notice that:

- You are affected by the energy and emotions of those around you.

- You are distressed when others are in pain.

- You are easily overstimulated and often left feeling overwhelmed.

- You have a hard time separating your feelings from the feelings of others.

- You take things personally and often assume that if anyone is feeling a little bit off, you've done something wrong.

- You need space and time alone away from others to refuel and recharge your batteries.

- You have a tendency to lean towards perfectionism.

- You don't fit in with society's expectations of what the norms are, based on the majority's behavior and standards of living.

For those of you who this resonates with, I can assure you that there is nothing wrong with you. To feel intensely is a strength, not a weakness. In fact, your sensitivity is your superpower. It means that you have greater levels of sensory perception, a keen sense, an innate ability to tap into the subtleties of everything and everyone around you. You may find that people often come to you for advice. Strangers tell you their life story. It's because:

- You are able to hold a safe space for others.

- You have a great depth of feeling and spiritual insight; your intuition is on point.

- You pick up on cues that others don't and can read in between the lines.

- You have a strong BS meter and can tell when someone is being inauthentic.

- You are incredibly artistic and extremely creative.

- You see beauty where most can't. You see extraordinary in the ordinary.

- You have a deep sense of gratitude for the simple blessings that others take for granted.

- You are a natural healer.

It took me many years to fully accept my highly sensitive nature as the gift that it truly is. I've come to realize that my ability to feel, sense, and read people is one of my biggest assets. That my sensitivity, my empathy, is a gift. It's my superpower.

So what's your superpower? What do people come to you for? What would be missing if you weren't around? It's likely you may have never really noticed your own superpower because it's what you do every day without even thinking about it. Many of us don't recognize our superpowers because they come so easily to us, so we don't think they're a big deal. We often take them for granted because we falsely believe that everyone else has these same capabilities, too. For example, maybe you have a natural ability to persuade others over to your point of view and inspire them into action. Not everyone can do this.

Many of us are unaware that we have people around us who look up to us for the skill sets we possess, so a good place to start identifying our strengths (our superpowers) is by getting some feedback.

- Fill Up Your Cup: Reach out to three to five people who you know will tell you the truth. Make sure they are people you respect for their contribution to the world, those you've done business with, people that know your true nature, your strong character, your talents, your abilities, and how you show up in the world. Ask them, "What is the one thing I do so well with such ease that it stuns people?" "What unique contribution do I bring to the plate?" You may have to dig a little deeper and let them in on why you are asking. Either way, take notes. What similarities do you notice? For example, they may say, " You're exceptional at building rapport and trust; people know that they can count on you." Someone else may say, "You accept everyone as they are; you're compassionate and nonjudgmental." Notice the common thread. Finally, now that you've gotten some positive feedback, make sure to keep these notes on hand so that you can access them anytime you need a reminder.

No matter your superpower, it's important that you practice moving from a place of trying to hide what you think are your flaws to embracing the very essence of them as the gifts that they are. So I invite you to:

- Call Out the Curse: What do you believe are the negative aspects of your special abilities? What has this experience been like for you up until this point of your life? Write these perceived flaws down in a bullet point list. Then take this list and…

- Flip It: Take whatever you thought was a curse and write out all the positive aspects to your special abilities. Be sure to notice any self-doubt, i.e., imposter syndrome that may creep in. We must be careful not to let our inner nemesis get in the way of unlocking our true potential. The purpose of this exercise is for you to recognize all the gifts that you may not readily see or allow yourself to acknowledge.

- Celebrate Your Greatness: Don't underestimate the significance of your origin story. Instead of being ashamed of where you've been, be proud of what you've overcome. Practice loving what you were once taught to hate. Embrace the gifts. What was once your shame is now a superpower, one of your greatest assets. Own it! It's time to celebrate your greatness and start focusing on your strengths, not your weaknesses. Be brave, envision, and imagine. What does your new life look like and feel like?

Almost every superhero story begins with trauma, a loss of some sort. It then progresses to a search for meaning and eventually to a life-changing moment—the realization of their superpowers. It's an inspiring tale, a journey filled with self-discovery and mastery. One of rebounding and rebuilding that gives us hope and the determination to keep going. Anytime we let our challenges make us stronger instead of weaker, we become a superhero. This means that any one of us can be a superhero by simply standing strong in the face of adversity.

Pushing Past Your Comfort Zone: Healing the Child Within

"If we can hold our vulnerability with a loving attention, the painful feelings can unfold and slowly move through us."
— MARK COLEMAN

Are you looking for a way out? When things don't turn out the way you plan, do you run and hide?

When we are in the midst of a difficult time, all we want is for the pain to go away. We want life to be less raw and more stable so that we can better cope. Sometimes the pain we feel gets so overwhelming we literally leave our bodies. We turn to addictions that act as distractions from the pain we don't want to feel.

When something traumatic happens in our childhood, oftentimes it gets buried beneath the surface someplace. As children, we don't have the tools needed to address these issues appropriately, so we develop coping mechanisms to survive. Unfortunately, we can carry these unhealthy patterns with us into adulthood, where they no longer serve yet continue to play out in our relationships. Hence why we can find ourselves getting triggered, reacting to people and situations as if we were still five years old.

Growing up with abuse in a time where we have little power over our lives can be traumatic, and trauma is known to affect us at a cellular level. I believe as a whole, on a collective level, we are dealing with mass trauma. Most of us were not taught how to deal with our emotions. We grew up with certain guidelines, definitions, and parameters. We were taught to shut down our emotions and were told that crying or getting upset wasn't okay. A good example is the belief that men don't cry. This belief has been passed down from generation to generation and still affects us today. This has left many of us emotionally constipated.

To top it off, our culture does a great job at distracting us. When we look to escape from hurtful situations in our life, we tend to redirect our energy and focus into another activity: smoking, drinking, gambling, shopping, eating, working, etc. These activities can become compulsive addictions. These addictions become a crutch, a false sense of security, a momentary fix. It's a way of keeping ourselves busy so we don't feel any pain. There is an immediacy of picturing somewhere comforting to go in an attempt to escape from the reality we are currently experiencing.

Within us there is a battle for control, a duality that emerges. Part of you knows the truth and part of you is in denial. We don't want to go through the storm, we just want to move right past it. We scramble for security. We get this queasy feeling and our minds run wild trying to find ways to save us from our own despair. Try as you may to avoid and ignore the problem, it still has a hold of you, for you are only masking the issue that you're not ready or willing to deal with.

Western medicine is a great example: pushing prescription drugs that act as a Band-Aid, causing side effects equal to or greater than the initial issue you are trying to address, and never truly addressing and getting down to the root cause of the problem. All it does is prolong the issue, all while keeping you disconnected from what's going on in your body even more. It's time to realize that doctors are people too and they don't have all the answers. You know your body better than anyone else, so it's important to pay attention to what your body is saying. This includes listening to our emotional body. We must become aware of our emotions as they lead us to becoming aware of our pain—what is working for us and what is not. The first step is to embrace any discomfort you feel, because this is where the magic happens.

When uncomfortable unresolved feelings come up, they are gifts asking for our attention. Your inner child is saying, "Pay attention! I'm anxious, I'm scared, and I need some love and affection." He or she is begging for you to listen so that you can fully heal. Your traumatized inner child is the underlying root cause of your self-sabotage, addictions, codependency, and more. Every form of pain we experience can be traced back to this part of us that simply wants to be acknowledged and held.

This is a journey of self-exploration and illumination. It requires us recognize when our ego is at play and curb our own judgments. It asks us to dig deep, to face our buried pain, and then see life through new eyes—through the eyes of a child:

- Mirror Work: Stand in front of the mirror and gaze into your own eyes. Keep looking. Stop criticizing yourself for a moment. What do you see in your own eyes? Is your inner child crying out for some love and affection? As you are looking into your own eyes, say to yourself, "I love you," "I forgive you," "You are safe." Most likely tears will flow...let them. Refrain from judging yourself. See and accept yourself as a perfect child of God. This is a very powerful exercise. I suggest journaling about your experience.

- Photo Therapy: Healing your inner child starts with seeing him/her again. You can't look into the mirror and see that little face anymore, but you can look at photographs. Find a picture of you when you were younger that you can access regularly. Ask your inner child when and why you think you adopted these coping mechanisms. How did they serve you then? Do these coping mechanisms still serve you now?

Your inner child at the center of your being is the most authentic part of you. It has the ability to transcend the confines of our adult egoic self. When doing this work, it's important not to shame ourselves, for our inner child already went through neglect. We need to learn how to re-parent ourselves, to be the mother and father we never had, to heal the child within. We must learn to embrace our vulnerability. In order to do this, we need to become aware of our pain points. We need to stop thinking our way out of problems and start feeling our way through them instead. Happiness can never be found outside of ourselves, and reaching for substances and thrilling experiences to numb our pain only provide temporary relief.

So I invite you to look at yourself in the mirror and face the truth. Take a stand and address your core issue, no matter what the addiction or circumstance. The next time you feel uncomfortable emotions arise and have the urge to reach for a fix, I ask you to pause, breathe, return to your body, and sit still with the pain. Push past your comfort zone and allow yourself to be vulnerable. Lean into it. Get comfortable with being uncomfortable. Practice the art of inquiry. Ask yourself why you are feeling this discomfort. Ask yourself what your body is trying to communicate to you. Have the courage to witness what it is you are feeling and then make a different choice, for the only way out is through.

Keeping It Real: The Key to Building Rapport & Trust

"We're often afraid of being vulnerable, but vulnerability creates genuine connection."

— GABBY BERNSTEIN

Did I mention I spent a whole summer in San Francisco homeless? Strangers lent me their car, trusted me to care for their pets, and left me for weeks at a time to look after their home and prized possessions. How did this happen, you ask?

People trust authentic people. Keeping it real and embracing your vulnerability drives trust. In order to be vulnerable, we need to feel safe. In order to feel safe, we have to trust. So the degree in which we trust influences how much we are willing to be vulnerable, and yet we must be vulnerable in order to build trust. It's a bit of a catch-22.

Trusting someone is risky; it is an act of faith. Building trust requires a willingness to open ourselves up to the potential of being hurt. We take an even bigger risk, however, in trusting ourselves—taking responsibility for our own well-being—and our ability to cope.

Oftentimes we fail to recognize how we distance ourselves from others, for what once worked to protect us from rejection in childhood is the very thing that now keeps us from the intimacy we crave. We're protected, yet disconnected. We hold onto certain beliefs that lead us to resist vulnerability, the very quality that makes connection possible. It's impossible to be intimate without vulnerability. This is how we form stronger bonds. Embracing vulnerability strengthens our relationships. There is nothing more daring than that which comes from embracing our vulnerability.

Allowing ourselves to be vulnerable is an act of courage. It shows strength of character and emotional intelligence. Vulnerability is highly underrated. It is not a weakness; it's a strength, a superpower. It means giving someone the benefit of the doubt. It means being honest in ways most people can't. It means that despite adversity, no matter how many times you get knocked down, you choose to get back up. You choose to weather the storm—not because you won't get knocked down again, but because you're not afraid anymore. Admitting you don't have all the answers makes you more approachable. Being vulnerable allows you to come from an authentic place instead of hiding behind a façade to appease others. This gives people around you permission to do the same, and because of this, they feel safer confiding in you.

Trust is one of the most important characteristics when it comes to discussing the aspects of influence. It is one of the highest forms of human motivation. In order for you to build rapport and trust with someone, in order to form a solid connection, you must first understand the four pillars of poise:

1. Presence: Presence is a state of being. It is the practice of being in the present moment. Cultivating the power of presence comes from creating the space to observe oneself. It is created through an acute awareness of one's thoughts, feelings, and emotions. It is a skill of observation and nonjudgment. It requires mindfulness, a keen sense to be able to tune into what is going on around us. It carries with it a silent power. It has the ability to draw people to you and open up doors. It's a person's ability to make their character known. It is the key to building relationships based on trust. Whether this comes naturally for you or not, every one of us can tap into and learn how to strengthen our presence.

2. Power: Power is a perception. In essence, it's the art of influence. It's the ability to create and produce a desired effect. A capacity to cause change. A willingness to act. It is relational. It's where our attention goes. It's what creates our reality. It is how we choose to respond in any given

situation. It's about winning the battles within ourselves. With it comes great responsibility—the responsibility to be aware of our choices and how they impact our lives.

3. Passion: Passion is a state of mind. It's the fire that burns brightly inside you. An intense conviction. A driving force that can be felt by those around you. It is the key to inspiring others. It energizes us and promotes contribution. It awakens our creativity and enthusiasm for life. It's contagious. It is what motivates others to come along for the ride. It creates discipline and enhances our focus, our desire to pursue excellence. As far as I'm concerned, a life without passion is a life unlived. So what are you passionate about?

4. Purpose: Purpose is our compass. It's the reason we journey forth. It's what gives us direction. It's what gets us out of bed every day and keeps us going. Having a purpose gives you the fuel to persevere and the ambition you need to make the necessary sacrifices to live the life you dream of. It makes it impossible to quit. It's having a servant's heart. It's a commitment to a cause, something meaningful and greater than yourself. As you begin to experience the joy of painting your bigger picture, you start to feel inspired by the determined, passionate, and impactful person you are becoming.

As you can see, each pillar is key to building a solid foundation of rapport and trust. So I invite you to shift your awareness in order to strengthen your foundation. Who are you being? Are you keeping it real? How are you showing up? Are you leading by example? Remember, the quality of our life is determined by the quality of our relationships—first with ourselves and then others. It all comes down to how well we are poised.

The Art of Influence: The Importance of Poise

"No quality is more attractive than poise—that deep sense of being at ease with yourself and the world."
— GOOD HOUSEKEEPING, SEPTEMBER 1947

Have you ever wondered how some people are able to grab your attention in an almost hypnotic way?

Poise can be hard to define. It is an unseen power, an intangible presence. It is an uplifting, peaceful, easy feeling that someone projects. When someone with poise walks into a room, you cannot help but notice their presence. The impact they have is evident. They often display that special something you can't quite put into words. They have what we call the "it" factor. They radiate a powerful magnetic energy. They are warm and welcoming and exude a sense of calm, a confident composure. This is because they are just being themselves. They are in alignment with their authentic self. They aren't afraid to be vulnerable, to show you who they truly are. They're not trying to prove anything to anyone. They are genuine. They are comfortable in their own skin. Therefore, they have the ability to influence those around them. Influence is the degree of actual change in another's attitudes, values, beliefs, or behaviors. It's an art. There's a grace to it.

Although it appears that some people just naturally possess this trait, it's actually a trait that develops over time. To learn to display poise, one must experience stress and then adapt. Think of bamboo. Its foundation is solid yet it sways with just the slightest breeze. It is flexible yet firmly rooted. Resilient and highly adaptable. It bends with the wind but doesn't break. In fact, it bounces back, unwavering in its strength even after the toughest of storms. Poise, in essence, is grace under pressure.

Somewhere amidst the storm, I was in charge of putting on a Global Summit catering to 125 key opinion leaders and doctors from all over the world. It was my job to coordinate and manage everything from preproduction (budget, negotiating contracts, and pricing with venues and vendors such as seminar space, audio-visual, banquet menu event orders, hotel rooming lists, florists, photographers, travel arrangements) to event execution (logistics planning, program management, delivering an overall outstanding event experience) to post-event follow-up (ensuring accurate and timely payments to sites and vendors). As you can see, there were a lot of intricate pieces and moving parts to handle leading up to and during this two-day event. Thankfully, I was able to coordinate much of this remotely from home and when the time came to be on site, I was armed and ready with what I needed to help get me through: B12 injections that I had stashed in my hotel fridge.

After the event had commenced, one of my colleagues made it a point to come up to me and say that they were thoroughly impressed at how gracefully I had handled myself during the whole process. I was surprised and yet thrilled to hear that feedback. I knew in that moment if I hadn't already gone through so much adversity in my life, I wouldn't have had the opportunity to practice handling multifaceted stressful situations like these with such grace.

Moral of the story: *Bend, don't break!* Remain open to being wielded. Don't be afraid to reinvent yourself and adapt. In order to minimize the impact of uncertainty, learn to see adversity through the lens of opportunity. In doing so, you'll become less overwhelmed by intermittent stressors and subsequent difficulties. You'll be poised for greatness! This makes a difference because when a stressor seems manageable, we perceive it as a positive challenge, which boosts our enthusiasm and energy.

So give yourself permission to be vulnerable. Align with your authentic self. Be honest. Be true. Be you. Dare to connect. Have the courage to show up and be seen. Unlock your true potential. Celebrate your greatness. Push past your comfort zone. Heal your inner child. Strengthen your foundation. Keep it real. Commit to living your life with more presence, power, passion, and purpose. Remember, we shut down possibility when we shun our vulnerability, so let us practice embracing it instead.

As author Elizabeth Gilbert so eloquently states, "Embrace the glorious mess that you are."

#5: RECLAIM YOUR POWER

"Ego says, once everything falls into place I'll find peace. Spirit says, find your peace and then everything will fall into place."
— MARIANNE WILLIAMSON

W hy is it that we allow others to affect our peace of mind? Maybe you've let your partner's bad mood ruin your day. Maybe you've let someone who cut you off in traffic get you really upset. Maybe you've let someone's criticism affect your self-worth. Maybe you've let someone's envy stop you from shining your light. Anytime we allow someone or something to have a negative influence over the way we think, feel, and behave, we are giving away our peace of mind, our power.

Growing up, my mom would often say, "Some things are not worth fighting for, pick your fights." At the time, I didn't understand; I felt compelled to fight against injustice. I saw this as a weakness on her part. But now I get it, now I see. What I thought to be weakness is in fact a huge strength. Fighting for what's right isn't as virtuous as we may deem it to be, for in doing so, we're engaging in a power struggle, emitting the same vibrational frequency that created the problem in the first place. We get to decide where we place our focus and what is worth our energy.

Many of us give away our power without even realizing it. Sometimes it's obvious, and other times it's so subtle it can be hard to recognize. Here are a few ways you might be giving away your power without knowing it:

- A Desire to Prove Someone Wrong: When you feel as if someone is doubting you, it can be tempting to want to prove them wrong. It's important to make sure we're acting of our own accord and not because we're trying to convince someone that we're more valuable than they're giving us credit for. We must be mindful of where we are placing our value. When we let go of the importance of what others think, we let go of the need to justify ourselves.

- Allowing Someone to Bring Out the Worst in You: More often than not, this happens in particular with those closest to you. Someone may push your buttons, triggering you to say and do things you wouldn't normally do. It's important to be mindful not to let outside circumstances control us and knock us off our center. When we are able to develop a sense of awareness and take responsibility for how we are showing up, we can then choose to break the chain of reactivity.

- A Lack of Boundaries: If you're feeling underappreciated and are finding yourself getting resentful, it's a sure sign you are giving your power away. It's important to practice stating our needs and setting clear boundaries. We must be careful not to lose ourselves in our quest for acceptance by saying yes to other people's requests when we know we shouldn't. When we have the courage to love ourselves enough to set boundaries, we know when to say enough is enough!

- Allowing Someone Else's Opinion to Dictate Your Self-Worth: Someone else's opinion of you is none of your business. It's important to find the strength within ourselves not to take things so personally and remind ourselves that what other people say and do is merely a projection. We need to be careful not to get so externally focused that we allow other people's judgments and perceptions of what they deem to be right or wrong dictate our worth. When we are immune to the opinions and actions of others, we won't fall victim to unnecessary suffering.

So the next time you're tempted to allow some outside source to sway or influence you, I invite you to turn your attention back to where it belongs. Peace must first come from within, and then our outer world will reflect it, not the other way around. So take your power back from your dependence on the external world by focusing on your inner landscape. Recognize where you have been placing your attention. How have you been giving away your power? How has the desire to be accepted by others interfered with your peace of mind?

Be mindful. We give power to what we focus on, so choose wisely. Take responsibility for your peace of mind by limiting your exposure to any type of heavy media content or negative conversations. Let go of comparisons and practice positive self-talk. If at any time you find your thoughts racing or your emotions heightened, consciously choose to redirect your attention. Look to things you do regularly that are not very mentally demanding. Take some deep breaths and tune into your body. Read a book, listen to some music or a relaxing podcast. Do some laundry, take a shower, or wash the dishes. Whatever it is you do, try to keep your focus solely on the task at hand. When your thoughts wander and you find yourself getting distracted, bring your attention back to what it is you're doing in the present moment. Focusing on basic tasks like these will give you peace of mind, at least for a little while.

Recognizing Codependency: The Need to Be Needed

"There is no problem outside of you that is superior to the power within you."

— BOB PROCTOR

Do you need to be needed? Do you find yourself taking on more than your share of responsibilities?

Although a sense of belonging and purpose is biologically ingrained within us, we must be careful not to become addicted to the need to be needed. This addiction is also known as codependency. How do you know if you're in a codependent relationship? If you have ever felt a compulsive need to help someone, at the expense of yourself, you have engaged in codependent behavior. In codependent relationships, we need to be needed. The underlying subconscious reasoning is, "if I fulfill your needs, then you'll never leave me." This type of exchange stems from a deep-seated fear of abandonment. It is an unconscious power struggle, a survival mechanism, a false sense of security. The need to control people and circumstances around us in order to feel safe and loveable.

It's been twenty plus years now, although it feels like just yesterday. I can see it so clearly. I had recently ended a relationship and recall my partner coming back to me in tears saying, "What am I going to do without you?" I remember in that moment thinking, "Oh my God, what have I done?" Is this what my ego wanted? The need to be needed. This validation as a confirmation in order to feel loved. In that very moment, I realized that I had unconsciously created this. I had somehow set it up so that someone needed me so badly. This was a pivotal moment in my life, as it shifted my whole perspective. It made me aware of the underlying subconscious programming that was running, the patterns and behaviors that I needed to shift.

There's nothing wrong with helping others. When we care for someone, it's natural to want to support them. However, it becomes a problem when we go too far, taking on their responsibilities as our own. It's not your job to play the role of the rescuer. It's not your job to be accountable for their actions. It's not your job to make someone else happy. Their problems are not yours to fix, yet some of us have a tendency to enable. When we enable someone, we do them a great disservice, as we take away their opportunity to learn from the consequences of their own actions. As hard as it may be to witness those we love suffering, sometimes it is necessary, as enabling can often make matters worse.

There's a fine line between helping someone and enabling them, and it's not always easy to distinguish between the two. When you're helping someone, you are providing assistance. When you're enabling someone, you are doing something for them that they should be doing themselves. Enabling can best be explained as supporting any problematic patterns of behavior that make it easier for that behavior to continue. For example, you threaten to kick your loved one out but fail to follow through. They act out in public and you end up apologizing, making excuses for their poor behavior. Perhaps you walk around on eggshells avoiding issues that need to be addressed out of fear that they will get angry. Maybe you end up cleaning up their mess for them. If you're missing out on things because you're so involved with taking care of someone else, then there's a chance you're enabling.

Most of us have no idea we are doing it. We go to help with the best of intentions, and end up enabling someone without even realizing it. In the process, we give away our power and we start to feel let down and taken advantage of. We have to be aware of doing this, because when we continually put others' needs before ours, it can get ugly. We get trapped in an unhealthy dynamic and this is where resentment and anger build. If we would only take care of ourselves as much as we are taking care of others, then all would be well.

We, however, are not taught this. Too often we seek outside ourselves for validation. Growing up invalidated in a chronically critical and negating environment can lead us to feel the need to constantly justify ourselves and prove ourselves worthy of love. Therefore, many of us get into relationships for the wrong reasons. We enter into them half of ourselves, seeking for someone else to fill the void within us. It's not conscious. Often we find ourselves participating in the same type of dysfunction we thought we had escaped from in our childhood, as we have a tendency to attract and engage in relationships that reinforce the wounded parts of ourselves—the parts that we ran away from in order to protect ourselves and survive.

Our parents may have tried their best, but they may not have had the emotional awareness and the skill sets to validate us enough. It's helpful to remember that they were probably coming from their own place of denial stemming from growing up in an environment where their deeply held feelings were invalidated in a similar way. This is yet another vicious cycle that is passed down and often repeated over and over again. As daunting as it may seem, it is possible to heal these wounds and fulfill our needs in healthy ways. We can overcome the hurt of invalidation and recover from codependency by re-parenting our inner child, developing authentic self-esteem, maintaining personal boundaries, and focusing on self-care practices.

So I invite you to take a good look around. Take some inventory on your life as it currently stands. At what point and in which way have you contributed to this type of codependent behavior? Which roles have you played? Be honest with yourself. Take responsibility and let go of the need to be needed, the need to control and fix things. Stop making excuses for others. Practice setting boundaries and following up on the consequences you set. This is no longer a time to enable, for those who are comfortable have no motivation to change their problematic behavior. Instead, empower them by helping them succeed on their own. Give them tools, teach them skills, show them how to access resources. In other words, give them the power to make their own choices and solve their own problems. Then focus on realigning and restructuring your own beliefs. What is the reflection you want to see? What kind of relationships do you want to have?

The Art of Self-Care: The Importance of Choosing You

"Self-care is how you take your power back."
— Lalah Delia

Do you have a tendency to put other people's needs before your own?

For a very long time, I was unsettled every time I'd hear a flight attendant's safety briefing: "Should the cabin lose pressure, oxygen masks will drop from the overhead bin. If you are traveling with children, please make sure to secure your mask first before assisting the child." I remember thinking, "hell no!" If I was traveling with a child, you can be damn sure I'd be putting their mask on before mine. And that statement says it all.

106

The innate desire to sacrifice one's own self to save the ones we love feels counterintuitive, as it goes against our natural instincts. Many of us stay in struggling relationships because we want to do right by those around us. We give and give without being sustained by oxygen. It's important to learn to balance out the loving care we give to those around us and the loving care we give to ourselves, for the act of saving one's own life first is what ultimately saves the lives of those around us.

Many of us have been taught to do good unto others, to give freely of ourselves, and we have a tendency to feel guilty when we put ourselves first. Often this can be taken out of proportion and used to downplay our own needs out of a fear of being judged and perceived as selfish. This is where self-care is often misunderstood. There's a big difference between being selfish and being self-loving. Anyone who tells you otherwise is unable to love themselves and is resentful of the fact that you are choosing to care for yourself. Self-care is not being narcissistic, overly confident, self-indulgent, or egotistical; it's loving yourself enough to allow your needs to be fully supported as well.

Self-care is prioritizing our own well-being, particularly in times of increased stress. It is about taking care of the little things that matter. It's about giving ourselves relief when we feel overwhelmed so that we don't lose ourselves in the madness of life. Self-care is any activity that we deliberately do in order to take care of our mental, emotional, physical, and spiritual health. It may look like taking a bath, a walk, or a nap, or taking time to meditate and reset in the middle of the day. It can mean taking care of the basics: making sure to stay hydrated and keeping your blood sugar up so that your body and mind stay energized throughout the day. It can mean limiting certain types of sensory input like avoiding florescent lights, harsh chemicals, loud noises, and large crowds. At times, it also means disappointing others, speaking your truth, setting boundaries, and walking away from toxic people in your life. The tough thing about self-care is there is no how-to formula. You have to listen to what your mind, body, and spirit need, and no one knows what that is better than you.

By no means, however, should self-care be a last-ditch effort, a desperate attempt to turn things around once you've already exhausted yourself and your reserves. One of my biggest lessons was the realization that I cannot give from an empty cup, leaving myself void and depleted. I learned very quickly that if I didn't get up and carve out a morning routine, then the mounting to-do lists would get in the way and I'd end up exhausted in serving everyone else but me. In learning to take care of my basic needs first, I am able to serve better, showing up with clarity of mind and a strong presence.

How you start your day determines how your day will go. So if you don't already have a morning routine in place, I highly suggest implementing one. Having a solid morning ritual is key to manifesting the life that you want. It's a great way to ground yourself, to ensure you start the day off on the right foot. It's the perfect time for you to practice creating healthy habits that boost your energy levels, increase your productivity, and promote your spiritual growth, well-being, and success. That being said, what does a healthy morning routine look like? And what steps can you take towards implementing one?

1. Plan Ahead: A healthy morning routine starts the night before by getting restful sleep. In order to get restful sleep, it often helps to write out your to-do list ahead of time so that everything weighing on your mind can get out of your head and you can rest easy.

2. Prioritize: Make room in your schedule. Set your alarm a little earlier so that you can incorporate a minimum of an extra ten minutes into your routine. If you have more time, I suggest carving out twenty, thirty, or even forty minutes. The good news is, once you get in the habit of doing this daily, you can adapt it to fit your needs, let's say, if you're traveling. The important thing to note is that it's not so much when you get up but how you get up that matters. That being said, I highly recommend you wait to check your email and news feed until after you've taken this time for yourself, otherwise the day will end up controlling you.

3. Create a Sacred Space: This can look like whatever you want it to look like. Any space that will allow you some quiet, uninterrupted time to reflect and focus in on your intentions for the day will work. It may help if you let your spouse, children, or roommates in on your scheduled morning routine if it is necessary.

4. Have a Conversation with God…the universe, your guides, your angels, or your higher self: Whatever your beliefs, begin with a grateful heart. Count your blessings.

Pray for the world, for your loved ones. Ask to be shown the way, to be aligned with the right people, places, things, opportunities, and resources. Be open to receiving guidance during your day for confirmation that you're on the right path.

5. Set Your Intentions: Focus on how you'd like your day to go. Take time to read and recite your empowering affirmations out loud. Meditate. Envision your perfect day. Do this in a way that you can see it clearly, but more importantly, feel the joy of what it feels like to be in the flow, to be on purpose, to be tapped in and turned on! Once you get the hang of this and start noticing the benefits it brings to your life, you'll never go without a morning routine again.

So I invite you to infuse your spirit. Recognize the importance of choosing you. As you go about your day, it's imperative you learn to carve out time for yourself. Practice putting into place daily self-care routines, if you haven't already. Manage your time by blocking out this time in your calendar, just like you would with any other meeting and appointment, for it can be tempting to skip your self-care in favor of activities you deem more important. Make sure to give yourself enough space in between tasks to catch your breath before attending to the needs of others, for you are no good to anyone if you are depleted. Remember, part of self-care is letting go of what's weighing you down. It all begins with having the courage to say no to others and yes to yourself.

The Power of No: Breaking the Habit of Self-Betrayal

"The first step to getting what you want is to have the courage to get rid of what you don't."

— Zig Ziglar

Have you ever said yes when you wanted to say no? Do you often feel obligated? Like the weight of the world is on your shoulders?

Many times we are taught to say yes to life, although owning our no is just as powerful, for it defines our boundaries and gives birth to integrity and respect.

It's important to discern our yes from our no and learn to separate where others end and where we begin. Sometimes when we have a decision to make we can feel torn, split apart between what's in our best interest and a feeling of obligation to another. In our minds, we conjure up these scenarios, trying to figure out how people will react to us. Our ego is making up all these stories and all these alternate endings, all the while projecting our feelings onto others. It's a never-ending circle that gets us nowhere.

Self-betrayal is a coping mechanism that many of us adopted early on in life, as it was once important to our survival. Many of us were taught to be nice through the example our parents and their parents before them set. We learned to consider other people's feelings before our own and that it was more important to keep the peace outside ourselves than to have peace within, which meant holding our tongue, putting up with people we didn't like, and even dimming our light. All to make others around us more comfortable and to spare us from disapproval. This is where we learned to abandon ourselves.

I've always had this burning fire inside me. On one side, it is what has fueled my desire, work ethic, drive, resilience; and on the other side, at times it has filled me with rage. I've had to ask myself many times over, "why am I so angry?" so that I could understand where this anger was coming from. I have come to find that the true root of my anger came from a subtle and easily missed form of self-betrayal. Being nice led me to betray myself in my relationships: staying longer than I should have, enduring abuse, and settling for less than what I deserved. It almost killed me. If I had taken better care of myself instead of worrying so much about others, I wouldn't have been so hurt, so angry. Somebody wasn't there for me…and that was myself!

I never had an easy time with this. This has been a lifelong lesson for me. Back in college, I used to say yes to everything and would find myself getting overwhelmed. I thought I could do it all. It took me a while to understand that I could not say yes to everything and, in turn, please everyone. I would have to practice saying no. As I started to practice the art of self-care, I began to turn down invitations that I did not resonate with, more specifically, family events that were considered obligations. Even though it didn't always land well and the guilt card was played on occasions, I had to be willing to risk disappointing others, as it was clear that my lack of boundaries was affecting my well-being.

At first, setting up boundaries was difficult, although they became easier to implement as my health declined even further, for by that time I had no choice. It's unfortunate that it had to come to that for me to learn this lesson. This journey taught me to acknowledge my own needs, to take back my power, to create boundaries, and to choose me. It taught me how to be my own health advocate. To truly listen to my intuition and my body's way of communicating. To love myself and remain steadfast in my truth despite outside judgments.

Breaking the habit of self-betrayal isn't easy. It takes time to recognize and replace conditioned patterns of behavior. It's important to become aware of how you are abandoning yourself and in what ways you tend to settle for less than you deserve. Living from an authentic space does not mean being combative. It means taking actions that are in alignment with who you are, not with who you think others want you to be. It means not compromising your moral compass for the fear of disapproval. Learning how to honor yourself is key. You must first honor, value, and respect yourself before you expect someone else to do the same. That being said, here are a few things you can do to help break the habit of self-betrayal:

1. Trust Your Gut Instincts: It's time to stop listening to others and trust yourself. There is power in your no. If your gut says no, then listen. The more you can learn to listen, the stronger you will become. You don't need to prove yourself. You don't need to explain your no, and you don't need a rational reason as to why you feel it. It's also okay to change your mind. Just trust your gut instincts and then act upon them.

2. Speak Your Truth: Don't be afraid to stand up for what you believe in. Honoring yourself means being upfront and honest about your wants, needs, and desires. It means

drawing a line in the sand with what you are willing and not willing to put up with. So practice speaking your truth one small step at a time, whether it's sharing an opinion you have that you would normally keep to yourself or just saying no. Over time, speaking your truth will build your confidence, gain you respect, and help you feel more empowered.

3. Set Healthy Boundaries: Every time you say no, you say yes to yourself. In order to experience fulfillment and well-being, we must learn to set boundaries. Healthy boundaries help us define our individuality, what we will and will not hold ourselves accountable for. They are a crucial part to our self-care. Boundaries are put in place to protect us, not to control others. It's not someone else's job to respond how you want them to. It's your job to respond in a proactive way that protects you from harm, in a way that keeps you from being reactive. Boundaries are set in place to limit how much you allow others to affect you. When we set a boundary, we are taking action by responding consciously. Setting healthy boundaries is not always easy, and standing up for yourself doesn't always look pretty.

4. Cut Ties: Sometimes we need to say no to some things in order to say yes to better things. We need to stop trying to fit a square peg into a round hole, dismissing those red flags and ignoring our intuition. We must realize that our frequency and vibration is not always going

to match up with everyone else's and that's okay. Not everyone is going to like us and that's okay, too! We must give ourselves permission to say no, wish people well, and be on our way. It's not about being harsh, it's about honoring ourselves and keeping ourselves healthy. It's about choosing who sits at your table. Realize that you're far better off loving from afar without doing yourself and the other people involved a disservice. Until we are able to say no and walk away from what doesn't serves us, we're unable to tap in to what does.

So I invite you to practice living in your truth proudly and firmly. Don't hide your here-and-now experience in the hopes of pleasing others. Express your truth and make a decision that best suits your needs that represents the life you want to lead. When in doubt, ask yourself how much longer are you willing to deny your own preferences to avoid confrontation. Look to see where you can practice setting healthy boundaries in your life. Have the courage to choose you despite the risk of disappointing others. I assure you the moment you do you will feel relieved. As you set boundaries and learn to honor yourself, you will blossom into the person you were meant to be.

Say What You Need to Say: Finding Your Voice

"Living out loud means having the courage to be exactly who you are without apology."
— IYANLA VANZANT

Do you say what you need to say? If not, why not? Do you often feel like you're walking on eggshells? Do you find yourself apologizing all the time?

Many of us are all too familiar with the expression children are to be seen and not heard. So we hold back in expressing ourselves because that's what we were taught. We hold back our true feelings for the sake of others. Our childhood disciplinary methods, whether reward or punishment, often have long-lasting effects that bleed into adulthood. Those of us who had parents that used love withdrawal as a form of discipline found ourselves conforming to expectation for the fear of abandonment.

When I was younger, my dad would often get angry and distance himself. Because of this dynamic, I found myself apologizing over and over again to win daddy's love and affection back. Fast forward fifteen years and little did I know that same pattern was still playing out in my young adult life. I had a roommate at the time who always wore a smile; he was one of the most easy-going men I have ever known. I remember the time he told me to stop apologizing. He had noticed that I had a tendency to say "I'm sorry" frequently and assured me there was no need for it and that all was well. This was another one of my big aha moments, when I realized that I had an unconscious coping mechanism playing out that was no longer needed to win over and keep the love and affection of those around me.

Moral of the story: *Happiness is an inside job.* It's not our job to conform to expectations in order to make others happy. Our attempts to say "just the right thing" won't shift someone else's unhappiness with themselves. Our peace of mind comes when we stop people pleasing and sacrificing ourselves to win approval; when we start living in our truth, in our integrity as our authentic self; when we learn to accept, love, and embrace all the parts of ourselves that we've kept hidden for so long.

So I invite you to tune in and reflect so that you may become that which needs nothing outside of yourself. Relinquish the quest for outside validation. Love yourself enough to tell others the truth about who you are. Catch yourself when you find yourself walking on eggshells and holding back. Ask yourself, "what is it that makes me hold back?" Stop seeking approval and worrying about what other people will think. Basing your self-worth on someone else's actions and words is recipe for disaster. You are responsible for your happiness, no one else. Let go of all the stories and beliefs that you thought were true. Remove someone else's control over you. Break the façade. Stop being who you think you should be and just be you. Choose to be respected over being liked. Find your voice, speak your truth, and have the courage to be who you are without apology. Say what you need to say even if the message does not align with the status quo. Repeat after me: "I will not stay silent so that others can stay comfortable."

Proactive vs. Reactive: The Heart of the Matter

"Every person's happiness is their own responsibility."
— ABRAHAM LINCOLN

Are you defensive? Do you treat simple questions as accusations? If so, you may be spending too much time on autopilot in the "reactive zone," a defensive state of mind.

Everyone gets defensive at times; it's human nature. However, when defensiveness reaches a boiling point in frequency and intensity, it can destroy relationships and damage personal and career success.

Defense mechanisms are part of our personal history. From our childhood on, they emerge as we learn to cope with stress, for better or for worse. It seems that when the going gets tough, they take on a life of their own, becoming a suit of armor to protect us. So what are some of your common defense mechanisms? Sarcasm perhaps? Rigidity, blaming, shaming, preaching, endless explaining, withdrawing into silence, loss of a sense of humor, all-or-nothing thinking? If you can't identify with any of these, denial may be your number-one defense mechanism.

These superiority-oriented responses are a cover-up for an inferiority feeling within that stems from a fear of rejection, a fear of being ostracized, and a feeling of inadequacy. So let's get down to the heart of the matter. What are your true feelings underneath the need to be reactive? In order to answer this question, we must be willing to tap into our emotions and acknowledge that we may be feeling hurt from what we perceive is being said. The world we experience and perceive with our five senses is a mere 1% of our reality, so our perception is a constructed reality. What this means is that our experience of pain includes a component that is constructed by our emotions and memories as well as by default functions in our brain that will automatically connect dots, whether this is warranted or not in a specific situation. Oftentimes we have a tendency to choose what we want to hear, and can therefore easily assume or read into what someone is saying.

One of the best ways to avoid being reactive is to take a step back and see things from an objective third party perspective. Seek to understand. For when we are truly listening with an open heart, there is no judgment to what is being said. If you are not sure you understand what the other party has said, just ask. It's important to repeat in your own words what you feel the other party has expressed so that you can be sure your understanding is correct. Don't say you understand when you have no clue, and don't apologize when you're not truly sorry. It's hypocritical. Nothing is worse than being on the receiving end of a half-assed insincere apology. This is yet another reactive coping mechanism developed in early childhood. Often as children we are made to apologize without fully understanding why.

Many people are not looking for an apology or an agreement on the issue at hand. What we are looking for is empathy—a safe place to be heard, to let it all hang out. So do your best not to assume. If you think you know what the other person is going to say next, hold off, for you might be wrong. Let them finish speaking before you begin to talk. And the same goes for you. Let yourself finish listening before you begin to speak. You can't really listen if you are busy thinking about what you want to say next. For when you do this, you are not fully present and the person you are communicating with will feel this.

Did you know that your heart generates an electromagnetic field that reaches several feet outside your body? This means that people who are in tune with themselves and those around them can feel you. Studies show that 60% to 65% of heart cells are actually neural cells that are identical to those in the brain, which indicates that the heart is a major center of intelligence. Understanding this is key in our ability to communicate effectively with others.

This means you can tell if someone's listening simply by scanning their energy. In order to do this, it will require you to notice the subtleties and nuances of your environment and those around you, for we communicate with more than just our words. Research shows that 60% to 90% of our communication is nonverbal. So if you are physically in front of someone, it's important to pay attention to the nonverbal clues such as eye contact, facial expressions, hand gestures, posture, and body language.

More often than not, it is easy to see if someone is in an open or closed-off positioning. For example, people who are open often have a relaxed posture, they communicate interest and show enthusiasm by keeping eye contact and making use of their hands. In contrast, people who are closed off may cross their arms and legs, avoid eye contact, and keep their hands close to their body. Being in tune with yourself and the nuances of your surroundings will help you get down to the heart of the matter.

Every day we are presented with opportunities to be reactive, to release that inner child who wants to throw a tantrum. Being proactive and recognizing our defenses can help us identify our reactive moments and become aware of them before damage is done. We must be mindful not to let what's going on externally shake our foundation. We can't control our external environment, but we can control what's going on inside us however challenging it may be. It's important to rise above the difficulties of the moment, see the big picture, take responsibility, and make the changes we need to make.

So the next time your personal warning system flashes "danger" and you find yourself reacting and getting defensive, I invite you to stop, tune in, and take your power back. Remember, we are not responsible for everything, we are only responsible for our response to everything. You know what pushes your buttons, so cut off your usual response at the pass. Instead of shooting a sarcastic comeback, ask a question to clarify. Instead of "brain dumping," shut up and listen. Lose your mind, open your heart, and actually hear what the other person is saying, not what your mind is interpreting. Choose to be proactive instead of reactive, minimize the damage, and begin again.

5 Steps to Reclaiming Your Power

Practice shifting your state daily and/or anytime during the week when fear, anger, or resistance pops up.

1. Pause: Slow down, take a few deep breaths, and bring yourself back to the present moment. Deliberately slowing down our automatic physiological fight-or-flight response is a sure-fire way to defuse any excess emotional distress.

2. Observe: Step outside of the heated situation for a moment and practice the art of mindfulness. Remain

neutral and refrain from judgment. Notice the thoughts and sensations that come up. As we observe, we get to decide how to respond, rather than be a slave to our survival instincts.

3. Witness: Acknowledge what you are feeling. Increase your tolerance for your emotional discomfort and lean into it. Give yourself permission to feel exactly as you do. Inquire. Reflect on your triggers: why you feel this way and how you might respond differently next time.

4. Expand: Shift your state, literally shake it off. Move your body in any way, shape, or form to help break down the excess fight-or-flight stress hormones and get your endorphins flowing. Go for a five-minute walk around the block or do some quick burst jumping jacks. Exercise calms the nervous system.

5. Release: Let it go and cut yourself some slack; self-deprecating thoughts only make matters worse. Catch yourself when the self-talk turns negative and consciously choose to shift it. Give yourself a do-over. Remember your why and visualize the outcome you desire as if it already exists.

In the wise words of author Shane Parish, "Just because we've lost our way doesn't mean that we are lost forever. In the end, it's not the failures that define us so much as how we respond."

#6: LIGHTEN UP

"Angels can fly because they take themselves lightly."
— Gilbert K. Chesterton

D o you take yourself too seriously? Are you able to laugh in the midst of your own awkward moments?

When we find ourselves facing unwelcome change, having someone tell us to lighten up is the last thing we want to hear. However, it may very well be what we need to hear. During times of uncertainty, it can be easy to contribute to a problem by taking ourselves too seriously. When life attempts to break our spirit, having a sense of humor is key to our survival, for where there is humor, fear cannot abide. Humor builds resiliency. It can help us keep going in times where it seems next to impossible. It can help us see difficult events as opportunities. It can help us get out of our own way long enough to see a way forward.

Here are some signs that you might be taking yourself too seriously:

- You can't take a joke, you take things personally and are easily offended.

- You care way too much about what other people think, and you wouldn't dream of putting yourself in a position where you could look silly.

I didn't participate in my normal routine that night. I got caught up on the phone in a long conversation with a friend as the summer sun was setting and didn't bother to get up to turn on any lights. I vaguely recall climbing into bed and onto my silk sheets only to scream and jump about twelve feet in the air in a matter of seconds. There I stood in excruciating pain in a state of delirium as shivers went down my spine trying to make sense of what looked like a very large, reddish-brown, medieval, gigantically grotesque creature crawl down the length of my queen-size bed. I quickly picked up the phone to call my landlords, who were a sweet Christian couple upstairs, and Roger answered. Unable to remove my hand from my crotch, I proceeded to explain to him what had happened. He asked me where I had been bit and I squeamishly explained, "in between." He then yelled out to Janet at the top of his lungs, "she was bit in the taint!" I almost fell over from sheer embarrassment. The next thing you know, Roger was downstairs armed with a butcher knife and quickly saved the day by decapitating the beast. Janet was quick to follow.

Side note: Did you know that centipedes don't stop moving just because you hack them up? Talk about a good lesson in resilience! These tropical creatures are built to last. They fight to the end, their pinchers still pinching for several minutes after their body is lying in pieces on the floor.

As you can imagine, it was quite the ordeal, the kind of situation where none of us knew whether we should laugh or cry. Of all the places to be bitten, are you kidding me? Somehow I managed to get through the night on ice, anti-inflammatories, and a couple of pain meds that Roger and Janet were kind enough to share.

The next day, I found myself in the doctor's office saying, "What's up, doc? This just taint right!" In that moment, finding humor against the odds allowed me to forget about the pain and embarrassment as I lay spread eagle on the exam table while they confirmed the fang marks and poisonous venom that the nine-inch-long, one-inch-wide Vietnamese centipede left in its wake.

For what seemed like months to follow, I couldn't quite put my mind at ease. Every time it was time for bed, I inspected it from top to bottom thoroughly before getting into it and then found myself tossing and turning while attempting to coax myself to sleep. The one thing I had going for me that allowed me to rest assured was knowing that my so-called incident was added to the list in the hall of shame as one of the rarest things that the doctors and nurses on staff had ever experienced. Talk about being the butt of a joke!

Needless to say, when I left Maui I took with me more than just a bag of macadamia nuts. I carried with me some unforgettable memories. Moral of the story: *Lighten up, and don't take yourself so seriously. No one else does!* Look for the humor amidst your darkest hours, for as the comedian Steve Allen once said, "Nothing is funnier than the unintended humor of reality."

Rekindling the Joy in Your Life: Laughter Is the Best Medicine

"Laughter sets the spirit free to move through even the most tragic circumstances."
— CAPTAIN GERALD COFFEE

Did you know that a good belly laugh can give you the same benefits as an aerobic workout?

Medical research is shedding a new light on the healing properties of laughter and its effect on our health. They say laughter is the best medicine: It boosts the immune system, decreases stress, lowers blood pressure, and reduces pain. It can also aid us in overcoming fear and has a beneficial effect on our overall well-being.

Laughter is one of the most powerful healing tools we have. It is the best form of therapy: a potent antidote to stress, pain, and conflict. Laughter helps us keep things in perspective. It is a tremendous resource for overcoming adversity. Laughter connects us. It enhances our relationships. Have you ever noticed how quickly people warm up to you when they hear you laugh? Laughter lifts our spirit. It lightens our burdens and inspires hope. Do you notice how much lighter everything feels after you laugh? Laughter brings us back to the simplicity of life and the joy that the moment can bring.

Unfortunately, as we grow older, our days can easily become a never-ending to-do list. Oftentimes, we don't even realize how far removed we are from experiencing spontaneous joy. We may find ourselves making excuses, saying that we don't have enough time, money, or energy to play, and yet playfulness is a wonderful investment that yields immediate results.

When we play, we have fun. When we have fun, we laugh. When we laugh, we relax. When we relax, we are more open to divine guidance and inspiration. When we are inspired, creative energy moves through us, and that's when we can manifest our desires. It is here in this present moment, in this joyful state, that we naturally attract wonderful people, situations, and opportunities to us.

So how often do you experience the joy of laughter? With so much power to heal, finding a way to add a healthy dose of laughter into our daily routine can make all the difference. In order to do this, it's important we find ways to reconnect to our joy, to find the humor in our day-to-day life.

- Spend Time with Your Pet: A great way to connect with our joy is through our pets. They are so present and in the moment. It's the little things they do that bring us joy. If you really pay attention, they have their own language, their own way of communicating with you. For all my dog lovers: They are the best teachers of unconditional love. Their sheer excitement for your presence as you walk through that door says it all.

- Play with a Kid/Play Like a Kid: Another way to connect with our joy is through children. Oftentimes, no matter how rough our day has been, just seeing kids at play can bring a smile to our face. So go remember what it was like. Ask your inner child what it feels like doing. Be creative. Choose an activity you haven't done in a while and go out and play. Be a kid, dare to dream again. Go have fun, go explore, have an adventure, get lost, connect with nature...laugh, sing, dance, celebrate, and find the beauty in life. Do whatever it is that brings you joy!

• Laugh at Yourself: Part of being able to find the humor in any given situation is having the ability to laugh at yourself. I can tell you from experience that it's unbearable to get through life without having a good sense of humor. Life is going to throw us curveballs. We are going to make mistakes. It's inevitable. And if we can't find humor in these seemingly ridiculous situations, we will live a good portion of our lives miserable. We must find the courage to let our guards down. To live with vulnerability and authenticity. When we finally let go of all the walls we have built up and they come crumbling down, what's left is the innocence and the pureness of our heart.

Once upon a time, amidst a moment of brain fog, I was headed out the door to do some errands. Without looking, I slipped my feet into some sandals and off I went. Somehow, it wasn't until midway through my day that I looked down at my feet and noticed I had two different flip-flops on. One tan one and the other pink with beads. For a split second, I stood there perplexed staring at my feet. How could I have not noticed? It's one thing to have two different pairs of socks on that no one else can see, and another to have two very distinctly different shoes on display. Although I've been known to have some fun with my style, this was a first! It was so noticeable that I was surprised no one had said something in passing. That's when I started cracking up…gut laughing! I couldn't leave the parking lot without taking a picture of the scene of the crime.

Looking back, there were times I took myself way too seriously. If it wasn't for all the obstacles in my path that gave me the opportunity to remain present, lighten up, and choose joy, I wouldn't have become the person I am today—a person who takes herself more lightly, makes people laugh, and is often described as having a quick wit and a good sense of humor.

Moral of the story: *A moment of laughter can make all the difference!* So rekindle the joy in your life by finding joy in the little things and laughter amidst the everyday moments.

The Bright Side: The Power of Positivity

"The pessimist complains about the wind. The optimist expects it to change. The leader adjusts the sails."
— JOHN MAXWELL

Do you lean toward optimism or pessimism? Is every setback just further proof that the world is out to get you? Or can you roll with the punches?

How you respond to life's ups and downs can say a great deal about you. Believe it or not, some scientists have theorized that there is an evolutionary advantage to optimism: Human beings may be programmed to view the world as just slightly better than it actually is in order to clearly recognize any real threats to our well-being and handle them appropriately. With an optimistic perspective, one is more likely to look for meaning in adversity and get a favorable outcome.

Let me clarify. I'm not talking about sunshine, lollipops, and rainbows here. Having a positive outlook on life does not mean we delude ourselves by ignoring or numbing out the harsh reality at hand. It means maintaining wellness by choosing to see the bright side of things: the possibilities and opportunities that are available to us. A positive outlook helps prepare us to take risks without being held back by bitterness or a fear of failure. Having the ability to rise above negative thinking while remaining realistic about temporary setbacks is a great strength. An enterprising optimistic person is one who sees opportunity no matter the circumstances.

Speaking of which, I'll never forget the day I met Carla. We were both laughing and cracking jokes in the doctor's office while getting our booze-less cocktails (high-dose intravenous vitamin c therapy). At the time, she was suffering with stage IV breast cancer, although you never would have known.

Measuring in at only four feet and eleven inches, Carla was a ball of fire, a go-getter, the life of the party. The holidays were her favorite time of year. She was always festively dressed and her home adorned and decked out to the hills with the appropriate decorations. Aside from hosting a haunted house out of her garage every year, she also hosted an annual St. Patrick's Day bar crawl in search of the best corned beef in town. Her vibrant energy amidst the pain she was suffering was an inspiration. She reminded me of me, with her smile, her light, her passion and spunk. A mirror as far as her spirit goes.

She was determined to beat cancer naturally without chemo, surgery, or radiation. And that she did, just less than a year after she was diagnosed. After hearing there was no cancer left anywhere in her body, she started building her cancer warrior club and was excited to share her health journey and story of recovery in hopes of helping others. This was about the last time I saw Carla, when she was in remission. My health had unexpectedly taken a turn for the worst that year, and so we lost touch. The next thing I knew, I was attending her funeral.

Come to find out during that time, she had stopped taking her supplements and getting her weekly treatments due to the high costs involved. Unfortunately, over a span of six to twelve months, she started having other major health-related issues and then the cancer came back with a vengeance.

For a good amount of time afterwards, I kept a picture of Carla bright eyed and smiling, celebrating and drinking a margarita— one of her favorite drinks—on my altar as a daily reminder to help me get through my darkest hours. To keep me on track and on purpose. To help me get up every day and continue the fight. To remind me to smile and find joy in the littlest things. To inspire me to see the light through all the darkness in order to pave the way for a brighter tomorrow.

Moral of the story: *We are responsible for our own happiness.* We manifest what we focus on, so we must be careful not to self-prophesize negativity, as it can adversely affect our health and well-being. Negativity feeds our fears and is self-defeating. It alters our perception and blinds us to possibilities. It blocks our good from coming in, keeps us stuck in a victim mentality, and can lead to hopelessness and despair.

Because our thoughts and feelings create chemical reactions in the body, our cells can become addicted to certain emotional states. That means whatever feelings we habitually nurse, we can become addicted to. Getting caught up in this feedback loop lowers our vibration, and when we reside at a low vibration we often attract people and circumstances that resonate at that same frequency. So it's important to keep a positive frame of mind as much as we're able, understanding that there is a greater good, a higher purpose playing out in our life even when it feels hurtful, painful, and confusing.

You never know when a window of opportunity is going to open wide. The question is: Will you be ready? When that window of opportunity opens up, will you be able to recognize it and take action? When faced with temporary setbacks, it is important to become flexible and adaptable without losing sight of our long-term goals. So keep your eyes open and your mind active. Be skilled enough, confident enough, creative enough, and disciplined enough to seize opportunities that present themselves, regardless of your circumstances, for every moment presents us with an opportunity to choose to see the bright side.

Breaking the Chains That Bind: Forgiveness & Setting Yourself Free

"Positive people are not positive because they've skated through life. They're positive because they've been through hell and decided not to live there anymore."
— MONA LISA NYMAN

What does it mean to forgive? How long can you punish someone? How long can you punish yourself?

The word "forgive" comes from the Greek word *aphiemi*, which means to let go, to release, to liberate, to set free. Simply put, forgiveness is a conscious choice, a decision to release feelings of resentment towards someone who has harmed us. It's letting go of our perception of what happened to us, the hope that it could have been different. In essence, it is a commitment to an internal state of well-being.

Many times we are unaware that we are the ones holding ourselves hostage. When someone we care about hurts us, we can choose to hold on to anger and resentment, or embrace forgiveness and move forward. Forgiveness might seem challenging at first because it's often misunderstood. Forgiving someone means you're choosing to let go of the hurt, to no longer dwell on what was said and done. It does not mean that you condone their behavior or allow it to continue. Forgiveness is about setting ourselves free. The moment we forgive, we release not only the situation and the person involved, but the pain we've been holding onto.

The act of forgiveness in its own right is incredibly powerful, as it has the capacity to heal and transform, although depending on the circumstances, it can seem almost next to impossible to forgive those who have wronged us. Here are a few tips that can help:

- Write a Letter: When things come up that are uncomfortable, it is best to find an avenue to release it. However, this is not always possible right away. So until a time can be set aside for clear verbal communication, it can be best to write a letter about how you are feeling. Take all the time you need to process and write this letter. Don't hold back. Write down how hurt you are, how resentful you are, how angry you are. This is a great opportunity for you to express and release anything that is bottled up inside you. This is a great exercise for letting go of any unresolved issues. If and when it's appropriate, by the time you end up communicating verbally to the other party directly, a lot of your pent-up emotions will be cleared and this will ensure a more productive, levelheaded, loving conversation.

- Transmute the Energy: In most cases, there is no need to send the letter; it is just a tool for your healing. A cathartic way to transmute these energies is to do a fire ceremony. Make sure to do this in a safe place; for example, over your sink. State your intention. For instance, "My intention is to forgive this person and let go of any and all unhealthy attachments to this situation." Then read your letter out loud. Once you've done that and processed all your emotions, tear or crumple up your letter and light the pages on fire. Release and let go. This is a simple yet powerful exercise.

- Walk a Mile in Someone Else's Shoes: Oftentimes, to let go of our deepest wounds, it helps if we see things from a different perspective. In order to do this, we must take a step back and step out of ourselves long enough to see the bigger picture. We must be willing to view the world in the third person, in an unbiased way. When we're able to look at the situation through someone else's eyes with a level of neutrality, curiosity, and compassion, we're able to see things in a different light. We're able to see what's driving someone's poor behavior. Without compassion, forgiveness is not possible. Forgiveness allows us to let go, and compassion allows us to move on with grace.

- Move On: You may have forgiven but not forgotten, and that's okay. If and when you catch yourself thinking about this issue again, gently remind yourself that you've moved on from the past, consciously shift your focus, and stop the suffering dead in its tracks. If need be, you can intend to cut any and all cords that remain that no longer serve you. Just visualize taking a samurai sword to swiftly cut away any remnants of the energetic cord.

Like any other skill, forgiveness takes practice. Just know that when there are things on your heart that you haven't forgiven, haven't released, like it or not they will continue to make their way to the surface in order to be seen and healed.

Many of us have layers of these emotions buried inside us stemming from some form of childhood neglect and/or abuse, as well as from a myriad of traumatic experiences in adulthood in which we may have felt powerless. One of these deep-seated underlying emotional issues that many of us struggle with is anger. Anger is our body's fundamental physiological response to a perceived threat. It's our way of protecting ourselves. The question is: Who are we really angry at?

Oftentimes we place anger outside ourselves to blame when the truth is we are really angry at ourselves, for not standing up for ourselves, for not listening to our intuition, for not trusting our gut instincts, and for playing the fool. As important as it is to forgive others, it is equally important to forgive ourselves. Forgiveness is the key to our happiness. It gives us the opportunity to recognize the truth and reclaim our power. That being said, here are three steps you can take towards self-forgiveness:

1. Accept Responsibility: Forgiving yourself does not mean letting yourself off the hook. If you've been making excuses or justifying your actions, it's time to accept your human frailty and admit to yourself what you have done. When we've done something wrong, it's normal to feel guilty and regretful about it. By taking responsibility and acknowledging that you have hurt someone, you can minimize negative self-sabotaging emotions such as shame.

2. Make Amends: Do this in person if possible. Own up to your mistakes. Express your remorse. Apologize. If for

some reason you're unable to have closure with a certain someone because they are no longer alive or no longer a part of your life, then it is important that you create the space for yourself, of your own accord, to release any pain and guilt; to express your remorse, prayers, and well-wishes in some way, shape, or form. Another great way to do this is to write an apology letter. This is important so you don't allow any toxic energy to eat away at you.

3. Learn from the Experience: To do this, it's first important to reflect, to understand why you behaved the way you did. Then, ask yourself what steps you can take to prevent the same behaviors from playing out again. Remember, people come into our lives to remind us how to love, to teach us something we need to learn. We are all mirrors of each other. The moment we look within and grasp the lesson, the closer we are to the light.

So I invite you to break free from the chains that bind. Say thank you to someone for reflecting back to you what you needed to see. Remember, each one of us is limited in giving love by the limits to our capacity to love. So forgive yourself, forgive your parents and anyone else in your life for being the only way they knew how to be, no matter how bad things may have been. Recognize that they were byproducts of their own parents' mistakes and flaws. Choose right now to have compassion, to love them as they are even if you don't understand them. Not because they apologized and acknowledged the pain that they caused you, but because you deserve peace. Lighten your load.

Let go of the fight. Open up your heart a little more and give yourself the peace that your soul is longing for.

Let us follow in the footsteps of hypnoanalyst Ryan Elliott, who said, "Forgive those who didn't know how to love you. They were teaching you how to love yourself."

#7: LIVE FOR TODAY

"Yesterday is history. Tomorrow is a mystery. Today is a gift. That is why it is called the present."

— ALICE MORSE EARLE

If you knew you were dying, how would you spend your time? What would you say to the people you loved? How would you live right now? If you died tomorrow, would you be pleased with the life you led? What would have been your contributions to the world? How would people remember you?

In these ever-shifting times, many of us are losing those that are dear to us. Our world seems to crumble when someone close to our heart suddenly passes away. Memories of the time you spent repeat in your mind. The ultimate sadness is in coming to terms with the fact that you are never going to see them again, hold them again, at least in this physical reality. The tangibility is gone. Therefore, the pain you feel can be deep and overwhelming. It's even worse when you find yourself wondering, "What if I had said this?" and "Maybe I should have done that?" Coulda, shoulda, woulda. It's a huge reality check!

Shortly after moving into a new home, I accidently received my neighbor's mail. So I went over to Mr. Hellman's to introduce myself. To my surprise, he was so happy to see me. You could tell he hadn't had any company in a while, as he was eager to connect. Richard was an older gentleman in his seventies, an avid smoker who suffered from COPD. Come to find out, he was in fact, alone and estranged from his family. So after our first encounter I made it a point to say hi as often as I could.

Every weekend, you'd see him out in his garage working on his model train set. Each time I walked by, I was taken back in time, to a scene set straight out of 1955. I felt like Marty McFly in Back to the Future catching a glimpse of something nostalgic. The guy clearly had style, and it was hard not to imagine what his life had been like. Aside from the cool train set, he had some neat pieces of art and a few stellar vintage signs hanging on the walls.

Speaking of walls, I could hear his TV blaring through the one that connected us on a daily basis. I recall I had gotten into another one of my disciplined work cycles and had left town for a day trip. Upon my return, I realized the TV wasn't blaring through the wall as usual. I have to admit it was all a bit of a blur. I had gotten so used to blocking out the sound of it that I didn't even know how long it had been off. So of course I got concerned. I knocked on his door, no response. I knew something just wasn't right, so I picked up the phone and started making calls to a few of the hospitals in the area to see if he had been admitted. Sure enough, I found out where he was and jumped in my car. I remember my heart was racing. I just wanted to be there so that he knew he wasn't alone, if only to bring a smile to his face.

Upon arrival, I was grilled thoroughly at check-in before I was allowed to go upstairs. I remember getting up to his room only to find out he wasn't there, and because I wasn't family, the nurse was unable to fill me in. I started heading towards the elevator feeling a sense of defeat with my head down and an empty pit in my stomach. Before I could reach for the buttons, I heard a voice call out to me. As I turned around, the head nurse on staff gave me that look. You know the one that says, "By law I'm not supposed to verbally share his whereabouts with you, but you should know that he has passed on." I kindly nodded, responding silently, and then turned to head home.

Tears started rolling down my face. I will never forget that day, the guilt I felt, that it was somehow my fault. If only I had gotten to him sooner, if only I had stepped away from my work long enough to be present, to notice any of the signs, maybe I could have prevented his death.

Moral of the story: *It's not forever, it's just for now, so don't wait till it's too late!* Take a look at the people who are on this journey with you and realize the importance that their presence brings in each and every part of your daily life. Reach out to them and express your heartfelt feelings, say the things you need to say. Don't let there be any ifs, ands, or buts about it. There are a million reasons but not a single excuse! Like the Nike commercial says, "Just do it!" We are not guaranteed a tomorrow, so today, start living every moment as if it were your last. What have you always wanted to do? Where have you always wanted to go? Well, what are you waiting for?

The Power of Presence: Doing vs. Being

"One of the most tragic things I know about human nature is that all of us tend to put off living. We are all dreaming of some magical rose garden over the horizon instead of enjoying the roses that are blooming outside our windows today."
— DALE CARNEGIE

What does it mean to be truly present? Why do we feel that we must always be in a state of doing? Are we afraid that if we slow down we might miss something?

It's actually the other way around. The truth is if we fail to slow down, then we are really missing out. How many times have you been in the same room as someone who was glued to their smartphone? Or someone who clearly didn't hear a word you just said because their mind was focused elsewhere? In this fast-paced world we live in, it's easy to get distracted. Our society has put so much emphasis on having an agenda that the value of our presence has been lost. We place such a high priority on "doing" that states of "being" are undervalued. We seem to have a blurred understanding of what it means to truly be present. If we aren't mindful of our presence, our relationships can suffer greatly. Every day, so many relationships are falling apart because of miscommunication and the lack of ability to really hear what the other party has to say.

Have you ever tried to express yourself and you know that you're not getting through? The other party has this blank stare on their face like they just heard you speaking Japanese. This can be very hurtful and frustrating for both parties, for communication is everything, and without it, we have nothing. In order to have a solid relationship with someone, we need to be able to tune into each other. In order to tune into each other, however, we must first take the time to tune into ourselves.

Slowing down is part of our fear. We don't always know what is buried underneath our masks, and so we are afraid to sit with ourselves in the silence for the fear of what might arise. When we slow down and simply observe what is happening in our lives, we can allow ourselves to witness all of our feelings. This forces us to get down and dirty, to peel away the old layers in order to make room for the new, like a snake shedding its skin. When you're tapping into your true essence, your core, it's not always a comfortable experience although always valuable. Try as you may, you can't avoid this process forever. You'll be amazed at what lies beneath all the noise and the chatter.

When I first moved to Maui back in July of 2007, a little over a year before falling ill, I was unable to sit on the beach without feeling lazy. I was burnt out, having spent the last year and a half building residual income and climbing to the top of a company ladder with the intention of positioning myself and those that I loved for long-term stability and freedom. It was clear I had become a workaholic. I didn't know how to fully relax in the stillness, in the silence.

As I went about my days, I noticed unlike the many cities I grew up in, nobody on the island was in a rush to get anywhere. Up until this point in my life, I had never experienced such presence before. I was blown away when strangers would ask me how I was, and it seemed they sincerely wanted to know. This is where I learned the power of presence, that presence is a state of being, not doing. I found that from this place of being, I could create and manifest even more, coming from a state that was effortless and not effortful. Little did I know this move would change my entire life.

Moral of the story: *We are human "beings," not human "doings!"* It's amazing what can happen when we take the time to slow down, to stop and smell the flowers. Life's too short, it's a precious gift, and we must take the time to relish in it.

The Time Is Now: Embracing the Present Moment

"The present moment is the pivotal point of power."
— DEBBIE FORD

Have you ever felt like there's just not enough time in the day to do all the things you need to do? What if there was no such thing as time? What if our perception of time has deceived us?

The key to being in the present moment is to redefine our concept of time. Time is defined as the indefinite continued progress of existence and events in the past, present, and future regarded as a whole. Our whole concept of time is an illusion. Linear time does not exist. Not in a horizontal sense anyway. If energy is always in flux, always in motion, then isn't it possible that time as we know it could exist vertically? The past, present, and future all coexisting together at once. If that's the case, then the only time we truly have is now.

Many of us get caught up in the everyday hustle and bustle. We are taught that it is up to us to "make it happen." This is where most of us lose ourselves. We have so much on our plates that our priorities get all turned around. We live in an age of distraction. Yet one of life's anomalies is that our future relies on our ability to focus and pay attention to the present moment. Life unfolds in the present, so living life full speed ahead on autopilot is no way to live. When we run ourselves ragged, we exhaust our options, our minds, and our bodies, and without our health, we truly have nothing.

Many of us seem to be searching for someplace else to go instead of being right here in the present moment. Often, we get so caught up in our thoughts about the past or the future that we forget to experience and enjoy what's happening right now. Our unhappiness, anger, and disappointment stem from thinking about events of our past. Our anxiety, fear, and worry come from thinking about the future, all of which we have no control over right now. So what's the use of worrying?

Throughout my health journey, there were many moments I caught myself saying, "I'm having the time of my life!" Because in that moment, I truly was having the time of my life. I wasn't promised a tomorrow. All I had was that moment. If I was up and out of bed and managed to get outside, it was a good day. Moral of the story: *The time is now.* So be here in this moment.

Despite what many people may assume, living in the present moment does not mean emptying your mind of all thoughts. It means focusing on whatever you are currently doing. It means being mindful. Mindfulness is a state of intentional attention. It requires awareness and acceptance. When we are mindful, we become an observer. You realize that you are not your thoughts and are able to go from moment to moment without judging them. Easier said than done. Like anything else, embracing the present moment takes practice. So how can we put mindfulness into practice in our day-to day life?

- Focus On Your Breath: Take a few minutes to take some deep breaths and just focus your mind on your inhaling and exhaling. This practice will interrupt any overthinking, curb your tendency to project into the future, as well as prevent you from thinking about what could have been. Focusing on your breath should help calm any anxiety and realign you with the present moment.

- Focus On the Task at Hand: Practice scaling down the greater scope, the larger view of things long enough to focus on what's right in front of you. Take things one step at a time. Break things down into bite-sized pieces so that you can gracefully manage and stay motivated. Focusing on the task at hand will ultimately help you be more productive, keeping you in the present moment and shifting any sense of overwhelm.

- Focus On Your Sensations: Consciously feel what your senses are bringing to your attention. Practice paying attention to what you see, smell, hear, taste, and touch. Observe, acknowledge, and accept what you're feeling in your mind and body without resisting or judging it. When you do this, any uncomfortable feelings and sensations often dissipate. This is a great tool to help you deal with your emotions and reactivity, as it should decrease the power they have over you. Focusing on your senses will get you out of your head and ground you back into the present moment.

So if you have been stuck in the rat race, I urge you to slow down enough to take some inventory. Take a deep breath and go within. Ask yourself how you can benefit from just being rather than doing. Expand your awareness and remain open to seeing things in a different light. Immerse yourself in the stillness. Who are you being in the quiet moments? Your presence carries with it a silent healing power that creates an intimate connection, for it's in the stillness that we find out who we really are.

As Maya Angelou put it, "Life is not measured by the number of breaths we take, but by the moments that take our breath away."

#8: ASK & YOU SHALL RECEIVE

"You get in life what you have the courage to ask for."
— OPRAH WINFREY

Do you have a hard time asking for help? Do you let your pride get in the way?

Learning to ask for help can be difficult for many of us. The simple task of making a statement such as "I need your help" can be excruciating. We all need help sometimes, although many of us have gotten into the habit of fending for ourselves. A strong desire for self-sufficiency can keep us from asking for the help we need. This, of course, is developed at a young age, another survival mechanism. Some of us may have had the experience of being let down repeatedly and so we do not trust that we will be met in our requests for support. We have developed the "if I don't do it, it won't get done" attitude. Can you relate?

For quite some time, I could not ask for help. In fact, I did everything on my own. I remember a time in my early twenties when I was sitting in front of someone I was doing business with and could not for the life of me ask for the help I needed. I was torn up inside. At the time, I felt that asking for help was a sign of weakness and I had this underlying belief that asking for help came with a price. How many of you believe this to be true?

Once again, this stems from the way we were raised, our inaccurate beliefs, and the lies we've been telling ourselves. Somewhere along the way, we may have bought into the idea that we should just know how to do things. Getting the help we need is fundamental to our development and success in this world. So it is important that we cast aside our self-defeating patterns of thinking and have the courage to believe what our mind thinks is impossible. We must be willing to go out on a limb and practice asking for the help we need. "Ask" being the key word here.

Here's yet another thing we can learn from our children. Don't they live by the principle that it never hurts to ask? We need to do the same. Why is it as we grow older, do we stop asking? It's mainly because we're afraid the person we are asking will say no. The fear of rejection gets in our way. But what do we have to lose? If someone says no, you are no worse off than where you started. But what if they say yes? We must be open to receiving in order to create and manifest the life that we desire, and being open to receiving means also being courageous enough to ask for help.

We may also be wary of asking for help due to the fear of there being strings attached. That by asking for help, we will somehow at some point be indebted to the other person. This most often stems from our interactions early on in life, where we may have been taught that asking for help is a transactional process, one that's laced with unspoken expectations. This type of exchange created a lack of trust, hence why we found it safer to rely on self, to handle things on our own. As a protective mechanism—to keep things more stable—we closed ourselves off to receiving so that we could ensure our safety and remain in control. This is why it may feel more comfortable to give, rather than to receive.

Another big reason why many of our questions often go unasked is due to the fear of burdening others. We can easily make the mistake of thinking that there's more harm in asking for help than not, and that couldn't be further from the truth. When we minimize our request before we even make an attempt, we deprive ourselves of the love, support, and care that we are so deserving of. Not to mention the opportunity for someone else to step up and into a role of service that can bring out the best in them. When we ask for help, we not only get our needs met but even more importantly, it offers us a chance to feel touched by another soul. If you are courageous enough to ask for help, you may just be pleasantly surprised at who is willing to help you.

Amidst all my travels, I've found that it was mere strangers who were some of the first people eager and ready to help. I vividly recall one of the first times I started to really practice and play with the power of asking. I had put most of my possessions into storage and was headed off to Hawaii with four overstuffed duffle bags and my guitar. This was around the time when all the airlines had started charging per checked bag on domestic flights and were getting pretty strict on their overweight charges. I remember checking in at the counter feeling a little overwhelmed in having to pay hundreds of dollars in excess fees I wasn't expecting and just asked outright if there was any chance they could waive the baggage fees. To my surprise, they were happy to!

Moral of the story: *Be careful what you ask for, because you just might get it!* If by chance someone is unable to give you what you ask for, it does not mean that you are not worthy. The answers to our prayers don't always show up exactly the way we envision them. They come in all different forms, shapes, and sizes, so it's important to stay open to the opportunities that show up. Being willing to ask can get you support with everything from help with the chores to a five-star review, landing another customer from a referral, a discount on a purchase, and even a room with a beautiful view. The possibilities are endless.

So I invite you to test the waters. Move through your fear of rejection, your fear of being a burden, your fear of being baited, hooked, and bound to someone. This is your chance to go out on a limb, let go of your pride, and practice asking for what you need; whether it's picking up the phone and reaching out to someone when you are vulnerable or being able to speak your truth and ask that your needs be met. Whatever the reason you're letting your needs go unmet matters. Here are a few tips to help you get started:

- Start by making a list of a few things you would like some help with and spend some time reflecting on what is stopping you from asking for help, or from taking others up on their offer to help. Do you feel worthy of the support? What are you afraid of? What is the cost of not asking for the help you need? What would you gain if you did?

• Ask someone if they'd be willing to assist you in running an errand, teaching you a certain skill, loaning you some money for your business, etc. In order to manifest our desires, we must be willing to ask for help. Whatever it is, you'll never know until you ask, so give it a go, you might just be surprised as to what shows up in your life. Make sure you're being direct though; people aren't mind readers, which brings me to another point…

• Take somebody up on their offer to help. How many times have you heard the statement "let me know if there's anything I can do to support you"? And how many times did you actually follow up? Many times people really don't know what you need or how they can be of assistance unless we are specific in our requests. I learned this the hard way when I became chronically ill. I made the mistake of thinking this statement was insincere and that's not the truth. More often than not, people are happy to help. Sometimes the best way to take someone up on their offer is to give them a specific task.

• Keep practicing. If you strike out, muster up the courage to try again. It may help to keep track of your attempts by journaling about how it played out so that you can continue to work through your fears and celebrate any positive shifts for the better. If all else fails and you feel like something's just got to give, pray to God and the universe or ask your higher self and angels for guidance. Ask to be shown the way. Just ask, and you shall receive.

All You Need Is Love: Increasing Your Capacity to Receive

"The greatest thing you'll ever learn is just to love, and be loved in return."

— DAVID BOWIE

How comfortable are you in receiving love? Do you feel worthy of the love of others?

Most of us are really good at giving love, but perhaps not so skilled in opening up and receiving it. Not being able to receive love is a major cause for many of the frustrations we face in relating with others. We are offered no greater opening to know the truth of who we truly are than in a relationship. Relationships are such powerful catalysts because they mirror the aspects we most need revealed for our soul's growth. What we see and react to in another we possess within ourselves. Abandonment, rejection, withdrawal—these kinds of fears prevent us from extending and receiving love, and they only cause us to reject and abandon ourselves. The only real pain we will ever feel stems from withholding our love.

So why is it so hard for some of us to receive love? To accept praise? Why do we get uncomfortable the moment we are positively recognized? It's because in some way, shape, or form we grew up in an environment where criticism was the default response. We also have an unspoken belief in our culture that says we are boasting if we give ourselves credit, and egotistical if we agree with any type of praise. We have been taught that it's prideful to think highly of ourselves, and this is why we have a hard time openly receiving compliments and all other expressions of love. Instead, we turn away from it, responding in all kinds of ways, not knowing that we are actually rejecting the very love that is being given to us. This lack of receptivity to praise can also be a reflection of our self-worth. It is known that we actively seek to verify our own perception of self, and so if we feel unworthy, we will feel uncomfortable when compliments are given—as praise conflicts with our existing belief system.

Our relationships can allow us to see the possibilities of what is left to be healed, if we let them. I can remember many years back one of my business partners complimenting me on a job well done, and at the time, I was unable to fully receive his gift. It was clear to him that his compliment wasn't well received and so he proceeded to express the importance of accepting praise for what it was worth. I will never forget that conversation, as it was a huge turning point for me in my life. I had become so used to going it alone, for fear of being let down, that I was scared of losing control, being vulnerable, and really opening up to receiving love. I was closing myself off to the love and support that I was really craving, and in turn, unbeknownst to me, it came across as dismissive to my colleague.

Moral of the story: *All you need is love.* Lacking the ability to accept praise at face value can have a negative effect on one's relationships, finances, and overall well-being. So it's important to take a good look at how we may be rejecting it.

- Notice How You Respond to Others: Do you deflect compliments when you get them? Do you downplay them, perhaps saying something to the extent of "oh, it's no big deal"? Do you qualify them by expressing how hard and long you worked? Do you feel the need to one-up or out-compliment the person giving the praise? Each time this happens, you're responding in a manner that says, "please don't show me love, I'm unable to receive it."

- Consider Why You Have a Hard Time Accepting Praise: What are you afraid of? Where does this fear, this limiting belief stem from? Does it stem from your upbringing? Maybe you haven't been praised often or had the opportunity to practice accepting compliments. Is it cultural in nature? Maybe you're afraid of being seen as vain. Or does it stem from your own feelings of unworthiness?

Once we are aware of how and why we reject love, we can work on opening ourselves up to receiving it. One of the ways we can do this is by working to improve our self-image. That being said, here are a few tips to help you increase your capacity to receive:

- Expand Your Vision: In order to increase our capacity to receive, we must stop looking at life through our rearview mirror—die to yesterday's illusions in order to be reborn. The problem is not one of supply, the problem is the size of our container. Our thinking is limited. Therefore, we must make a conscious choice to move past our limitations, challenge our beliefs, and expand our vision in order to see clearly. We must make room, clear the clutter, and stretch our thinking by believing something we previously thought was impossible. Once we make room for love, for positive reinforcement, for prosperity, God will show off and the universe will provide in the most unexpected ways.

- Let Go of Comparisons: Comparing ourselves to others is an unnecessary and unkind way to measure our worth. Our self-worth isn't dependent on what anyone else has, says, or does. While it may seem that everyone on social media is living their best life, it's important to remind ourselves that we're only seeing the highlight reels. Often, we have no idea what's really going on behind the scenes and chances are it's a lot messier than what the photoshopped filters portray. So bring your focus back to yourself. Instead of comparing yourself to someone else's accomplishments, try looking at how you're doing in comparison to who you were last month or last year and make sure to give yourself credit where credit is due.

- Surround Yourself with Positive Associations: It's important to align yourself with those who have been where you want to go: the doers, the visionaries, the dreamers. Those who think outside the box. Those who know what is possible, for you can't discuss achieving your goals with those who don't have any. It's important we surround ourselves with those that are equally yoked, those who can reflect back to us the truth of who it is we are.

- Create a Culture of Praise: A great way we can practice being more accepting of praise is to encourage and celebrate others—to lift up those around us by giving out genuine compliments, for it's important for all of us to know just how special we are to each other. A simple compliment can make a big difference, not only on the receiving end but also for the giver. Compliments are gifts of love; they amplify positivity and satisfy our fundamental biological need to be recognized, seen, and appreciated by others.

So the next time someone gives you a compliment, I invite you to allow yourself to be positively recognized—to be loved and appreciated for what you bring to the table. Practice retraining yourself by expressing gratitude. Remind yourself that there is no need to deflect, downplay, or qualify the praise that is given. Simply smile and say thank you. Accept compliments as the gifts that they are and open yourself up to receiving love by giving others the gift of loving you.

Trust In Your Inner Knowing: Let Your Intuition Be Your Guide

"Trust your inner guidance to reveal to you whatever it is you need to know."

— LOUISE HAY

Are you in need of some guidance, some assistance to point you in the right direction? If you are, who do you turn to? A friend or family member perhaps?

Many times we tend to go outside ourselves in seek of the answer, as it may feel more comfortable, more safe following someone else's guidance. Just keep in mind, though, that those who offer you advice may not know the full picture of everything that you need to take into consideration when making the decision of what is best for you, and not everyone has your best interest at heart. You are the only one that knows what's best for you. That being said, there's a higher source of guidance within us to tap into. It's called our intuition. It's our spiritual wisdom, an instinctive feeling, an inner knowing, the ability to acquire knowledge without conscious reasoning, and it can play a big role in guiding us in the right direction. Our intuition is an internal GPS, our inner compass. It can help us get clear about where we are, where we want to go, and the best route to get there.

One of the important aspects of tapping into our intuition is understanding the power of discernment. Discernment can help us recognize where we are on the map in order to use our intuition and navigate accordingly. Discernment is the process of making distinctions in our thinking about truth. It is the ability to have keen insight, a deep understanding. Our ability to discern is fundamental when making decisions. Anytime we need to make an important decision that can have a profound impact on our life, it's important to go within for the answer and let our intuition be our guide.

1. Ground Yourself: Sometimes it's as simple as getting out in nature and taking a walk to get some fresh air, move our body, and release any stuck energy. If we are not present, grounded, and centered, our guidance can be hard to hear.

2. Be Patient: Relax your mind and open your heart. Ask for guidance and listen for the response. You may not receive an answer immediately. Your guidance will most likely find you when you least expect it.

3. Take a Step Back: Sometimes we need to take a step back in order to move forward and place our focus elsewhere. It's a catch-22, for when we seem to need guidance the most is when we often have trouble hearing the answer. On this journey we call life, it's important to set our intentions and give it our all. However, it's not always about pushing forward; sometimes the more we push, the worse it gets. We need to know when to back off, when to surrender and wait for the call. We've all heard the saying timing is everything, so sensing the timing of things is important when making our decisions.

There seems to be somewhat of a misconception around how our intuition communicates with us. Many people make the mistake of believing that our intuition stems from our emotions and therefore can be unreliable. Because our intuition is sourced from our higher self, it has no emotional charge; it is neutral. Just like learning any language, it takes time to practice tuning into our intuition and its subtle way of communicating to us. When things are unclear and you're not sure which direction to go, it helps to:

Pay Attention to What's Going On around You

It's important to pay attention to signs and synchronicities, as they can show up in many different forms: through your dreams, through the words someone says. For instance, you may overhear a conversation between passersby that appears to address your question at hand. Or out of the blue, you might start singing a song that pops into your head and next thing you know that very same song is suddenly playing on the radio. More often than not, there is a message for you in that song. Perhaps an unexpected video pops up in your news feed that gives you some pertinent information related to a project you're working on.

You may get signs through symbols, pictures, or just a deep knowing. For example, you could come across an animal or an insect that had deep meaning to a passed-on loved one. This could be a sign that they are looking after you and trying to communicate with you. There could literally be a sign on the road trying to get your attention or a car that cuts you off with a license plate or bumper sticker that pertains to something personal and meaningful to you. More often than not, synchronicities are a sure sign that you are on the right path.

Listen to That Little Voice Inside Your Head

You know, the one that said not to take the freeway today. Often it's just a passing thought that can help guide us towards a big breakthrough and even help us avert disaster.

Sometimes a certain sequence of events will get rearranged to shift our daily routine for the better. For instance, have you ever been heading somewhere and had a sudden urge to stop at a place that you didn't plan on, only to run into an old friend? Maybe this friend had some information to share with you that turned out to be exactly what you needed. If you hadn't listened to your intuition, you would have never run into that old friend and received the news.

This voice—our intuition—can often be but a whisper, and so it can be easy to brush it off. We may choose to override it consciously or unconsciously. Either way, when we doubt our higher self, we give power to our doubt. One of the best ways to curb self-doubt and begin to trust in our intuition is by looking back and recalling the times when we ignored it. When we know things would have gone differently if we had heeded the advice. This is a good reminder that there are higher forces at work guiding us through our day.

Focus On the Sensations You Feel in Your Body

It's important to learn how to listen to our body so that we can accurately tune into our gut instincts to help us discern fact from fiction. Once we get clear on how the truth feels, we will be able to identify the difference and our ability to discern will be greatly enhanced. Instead of making decisions based in fear and our past conditioning, we can make decisions based in wisdom that is in alignment with our highest good.

I must admit, somewhere along the way, in my commitment to being nonjudgmental, I failed at times to be appropriately discerning. I found myself stuck in a confused state, between what I was intuitively feeling and what someone else was portraying. Through all my trials and tribulations, I've come to realize that it's either a "hell yes!" or a "no." I've learned that hanging out in the land of "maybe" is where we can get ourselves in trouble. It's best to follow what lights us up. If it doesn't feel right, then most likely it isn't.

For example, how many times have you ignored your intuition only to create your own heartbreak? All too often, those of us who tend to see the good in others ignore the red flags that are trying to get our attention that keep us out of harm's way. If something doesn't feel right, you know it. It's called your gut instinct. Our gut instinct is our primal wisdom, and its purpose is to protect us. Gut instincts are often spontaneous and seem to come out of the blue. You may experience anxiety, nausea, full-body chills, sudden hypervigilance, a feeling of dread, or a strong urge to do something. If you do, whatever your beliefs, don't question it. Remove yourself from the situation. This is your body's way of communicating to you. It's trying to get your attention. So trust yourself and have the confidence to act upon it.

When you learn to pay attention to all the signs, synchronicities, hunches, and whispers, you're able to bypass obstacles in your life. If something or someone seems out of place, doesn't feel right, or stands out like a sore thumb, let it go. That's what you created then, this is now, and it's a whole new world!

As you learn to open your heart, listen, and trust more, you will find many doors opening, opportunities presenting themselves, and what seem like magical events taking place. So I invite you to trust in your inner knowing. Go beyond the self-doubt, letdowns, and disappointments. Find peace inside of you despite adversity. Instead, ask for a sign. Ask your higher self, ask your angels, ask God, "How can I learn from this?" Then let go of your mind and follow your heart. Heed the call. Pay attention to how your body feels. Allow your intuition to lead you in the right direction, to show you the way.

As Jesus states in his Sermon on the Mount, "Ask and you shall receive, seek and you shall find, knock and the door shall be answered."

#9: HAVE FAITH WHATEVER
IT TAKES

"When you have come to the edge of all light that you know, and are about to drop off into the darkness of the unknown, faith is knowing one of two things will happen: There will be something solid to stand on, or you will be taught to fly."

— PATRICK OVERTON

———————

What does it mean to have faith? Faith is a belief in the trustworthiness of an idea that has not been proven. It's walking the blind path, believing in what we cannot see and doing it anyway. According to Martin Luther King, "Faith is taking the first step, even if you don't see the whole staircase."

There is something to be said about having faith. I don't mean in a religious sense, but overall. We must tap into the courage that lies within and find the strength to face our fears head on. You can't run away from them, you can't walk around them, the only way out is through.

A couple years after the 2008 recession hit, somewhere in the early stages of my health journey, I came home just in time to find my parents' relationship unraveling. After losing the business I had worked so hard to build, I had no choice but to leave my residence in Hawaii. It seemed like just yesterday I was leaving my parents' house, heading off to college excited about my future and newfound freedom, only to find myself back at home fifteen years later. I remember feeling so defeated, barely able to look my father in the eye. Although grateful to have a roof over my head, I felt that it was far from the safe haven I needed to heal and recover.

One night, the three of us went out to dinner. My mom, wrought with pain, blatantly blamed me in the middle of a crowded restaurant that my presence was the reason why their relationship was currently failing. I can remember shrinking, the sting of her words cutting so deep, like somehow it was all my fault that I got so sick and had no choice but to crawl back home for some temporary refuge. To say that I was in shock was an understatement; the pain I felt was overbearing at the time. I remember getting up from the table and walking out of the restaurant into the alleyway, my back against the wall sliding down onto the ground in a puddle of tears, watching the cars go by out of the corner of my eye feeling like it was the end of the world.

In that moment and for some time to follow, I felt empty and alone, trapped not knowing where to go and how to move forward. The next day, I packed up my stuff, borrowed a friend's car while I slept on another friend's couch, and spent the next couple weeks soul searching and researching my options. I had just enough money left in my bank account to buy a one-way ticket to San Francisco. What was in San Francisco, you ask? Well, I was about to find out.

As I made my way out of the San Francisco airport, I was picked up by a middle-aged woman in a Prius who I didn't know. Through a friend of mine, I had heard that she was in need of some assistance selling her five-million-dollar home in northern Marin County. At the time, she was going through a divorce and I had agreed to help her sell items on Craigslist, along with staging the house for sale in exchange for room and board. This was a first for me. Talk about starting over. Once again, I showed up with my laptop, two suitcases, and my guitar. Aside from that, all I had was my relationship-building and networking skills. I thought that going to this major hub of a city could help me start a new life amidst the economic turndown, as Las Vegas still hadn't recovered.

Although Novato was much farther out from San Francisco than I had hoped it to be, I needed to buy some time in order to figure out my next steps. At first, it seemed we had really hit it off, although as time went by I felt I was being taken advantage of tending to tasks above and beyond the scope of what we had initially discussed. I started to feel more like a live-in maid and less than a friend of a friend helping someone in transition. I thought we were on the same page regarding our agreement, as I had made sure to discuss her expectations beforehand while also stating my needs and making clear that I would be spending half my days rebuilding my business. I never in my wildest dreams thought I'd find myself in the middle of a Disney movie playing the part of Cinderella, feeling as if I had no way of escaping what had become a bit of a nightmare.

The time I spent in the Bay Area was all about having unwavering faith. There I was again, not sure of which way to go and how to move forward; there was no roadmap. All I knew was that I had to move, even if I didn't know where to go.

It took a lot of strength to let go and walk the blind path. It wasn't easy being on-the-go during my time of illness without a car and a stable roof over my head. In order to move forward, I had to have faith; I had to have insight. I had to be willing to think outside the box, try something new. I had to pray and ask to be shown the way. In doing so, I was led on a great adventure. To my surprise, I ended up in yet another multimillion-dollar home. This time, I was pet sitting in the Berkeley Hills, alone and in peace, able to do my work while taking in the breathtaking, spectacular views of the East Bay.

Moral of the story: *Keep the faith.* When you feel like things are falling apart and there is no solid ground to stand on, take a leap of faith, put one foot in front of the other, and have the courage to venture into the unknown. Trust that the path will unfold in front of you with every step you take. What may seem like a challenge is exactly what's guiding you to where your supposed to be. Remember, things don't happen by accident or by chance. There's something greater unfolding going on behind the scenes that's bigger than what you're able to see right now. So trust that you'll be given wings to fly. You don't need to know the how, just remember your why. Surrender, lean into it, and have faith in the process. Believe in something bigger than yourself. Have faith in God and the powers that be, but most of all have faith in yourself. It takes strength to keep showing up anyway amidst the uncertainty. Take it one step at a time, believe in miracles, and no matter what happens, keep the faith!

Three Feet from Gold: The Power of Perseverance

"One of the most common causes of failure is the habit of quitting when one is overtaken by temporary defeat."
— NAPOLEON HILL

Do you give up at the first sign of opposition?

More than five hundred of the most successful men this country has ever known told Napoleon Hill—the author of *Think and Grow Rich*—that their greatest success came just one step beyond the point at which defeat had overtaken them. One of the stories in this book is about a man named Darby, who many years ago went to Colorado during the gold rush to find his fortune. He staked his claim, bought a pick and a shovel, and went to work. After weeks of digging, he struck gold! When this happened, he decided to go borrow some money from friends and family to purchase the necessary machinery to finish the job. In doing so, he managed to get the first load of gold to pay off his debt and now he was ready for the profits. Then something happened. The vein of gold had disappeared. He desperately kept drilling, and after many failed attempts, he decided to quit. He sold the machinery to a junkman for a few hundred dollars and went back home.

Little did he know the junkman had called in an engineer to do a little calculating. The engineer discovered that the project had failed because Darby was not familiar with "fault lines." His calculations showed that the gold vein would be found just three feet away. Long story short, the junkman ended up taking millions of dollars of gold from the mine, as he knew enough to seek expert advice before giving up.

Moral of the story: *If at first you don't succeed, try and then try again.* Don't give up at the first sign of opposition, for defeat is only temporary. It's an opportunity to discover what went wrong. Those that are considered successful have fallen down many times. The only difference is, they got back up and did it all over again.

Get In the Game: The Art of Resilience

"Obstacles do not block the path, they are the path."
— Zen Proverb

How resilient are you? Are you able to face life's difficulties head-on? Are you really in the game? Or are you just watching from the sidelines?

Perhaps you're feeling tattered and torn, tired of your many failed attempts. Have you ever noticed that when a child wants something, they are relentless? Being relentless means not giving up. It means being steadfast when pursuing your goals, even if others don't get it. If Dad says no, they go ask Mom. They're persistent. They keep at it even when the going gets tough! Persistence is a quiet resilience that keeps us moving forward despite difficulty.

Children teach us that if you really want something, you have to be willing to go above and beyond the first initial defeat. You must be willing to fully commit. How do they do this? Is it their desire, or strong willpower perhaps? The fact that they're too young to be tired and jaded? What is it that keeps them going? Oftentimes, it's an unbeatable combination of resilience and perseverance.

Resilience is a state of being. It's the ability to withstand adversity, adapt to difficult situations, and bounce back. It's a reservoir of strength we can call on in times of need to carry us through. Resilient people experience problems just like everyone else. The difference is, they persevere. They perceive hard times as temporary, choosing not to let their circumstances define them. Perseverance is a state of mind. It's not giving up. It's about being disciplined and determined. It means having faith when adversity is knocking at your door.

We've all heard the phrase when one door closes, another one opens. That's because we closed one door before we opened another. So why is it that we seem to think that we can hold one door open as we open another? Let's take a job for instance. Most people say that before you let go of one job, you had better have another one lined up to take its place. We say this because we want stability, a comfortable safe place to land. But there are no guarantees in life. Playing it safe is not really playing at all. Sometimes we just have to jump.

The road to resilience is often paved with stress and strain. The more challenges we face, struggle with, and conquer, the more resilient we become. Obstacles are a part of this game called life. Some are overcome easily, while others seem insurmountable. When these seemingly insurmountable obstacles arise, it can be easy to lose sight of our goals, our dreams, our worth, and our value. Right now, many of us are fearing for the lives of ourselves and our loved ones. Many of us are grieving the life we once had. When we go through hard times like these, it's easy to feel overwhelmed, unsure, isolated, and lonely. During such times, it helps to remind ourselves that there is no wasted experience, for within these difficulties that we encounter are lessons to be learned. The obstacles on our path are merely a means to self-discovery.

When we are resilient, nothing can hold us back. That being said, in order to help us cultivate a belief in our ability to cope, we must focus on things that are not dependent on other people or outside circumstances. We need to know we have what it takes inside us to get through this. Therefore, it's important to develop our strength of character so that we can harness the best of us when we need it the most. We need to believe in our own abilities, to feel confident that there is a well of strength within us to draw upon in order to navigate these uncharted waters.

Throughout this book, we've touched upon a variety of attributes that can help us maximize our resiliency during hardship. Some of these key factors include: having a positive attitude, the willingness to witness and regulate emotions, and the ability to see failure as a form of helpful feedback. Here is a more detailed list of what I refer to as the twenty-three qualities of a spiritual warrior. A spiritual warrior is a person who is self-aware, who challenges their beliefs, and who faces their fears.

They lead by example, using adversity as their compass. They recognize the battle that's taking place between their head and their hearts, and seek to bridge that gap daily. Spiritual warriors are willing to do whatever it takes, no matter how hard it may be.

1. Awareness: a conscious knowledge of one's character, feelings, motives, and desires. The ability to see clearly and objectively through reflection and introspection.

2. Adaptability: an ability to pivot, to adjust to change. To be flexible to one's environment.

3. Accountability: taking responsibility. Following through. Doing what you say you will do.

4. Ambition: an insatiable hunger. A compulsion to excel. Passionate and highly motivated.

5. Authenticity: being genuine, real, and true. Actions that are congruent with your core values and beliefs.

6. Commitment: an agreement to do something. Dedication to a cause. Fulfilling an intention.

7. Compassion: emotional intelligence. Being perceptive and sensitive to the needs of others. The ability to walk a mile in someone else's shoes. An understanding of someone else's pain and the desire to alleviate it.

8. Confidence: belief in oneself. Strength of conviction. Willingness to act accordingly. Trusting in yourself and your inner knowing.

9. Courage: having the strength to face your fears head on. The willingness to confront pain and uncertainty. Acting on convictions and speaking up in spite of opposition. The ability to take a leap of faith and venture into the unknown.

10. Curiosity: a desire for knowledge, an inquisitiveness. Aspires to seek the truth. Questions their beliefs and preconceived notions.

11. Discipline: a controlled behavior. Consistency of action. The ability to regulate, to follow through on your commitments. Doing what you know you should do even when you don't feel like it.

12. Faith: a belief in the trustworthiness of an idea that has not been proven. A strong conviction. Having confidence in someone or something. Believing in something bigger than yourself. Trusting that you are divinely guided.

13. Fortitude: a strength of mind, mentally and emotionally, that enables courage in the face of adversity.

14. Humility: the quality of being humble. The ability to keep your ego in check. To acknowledge your shortcomings. Having the strength to admit that you don't have all the answers. A willingness to serve without expectation of reward or recognition.

15. Humor: the capacity to perceive and express what is funny. The ability to laugh at yourself and your situation.

16. Integrity: a steadfast adherence to moral principles. The ability to be honest. Doing what is right even when no one is watching.

17. Mindfulness: the practice of bringing one's attention to the present moment. An ability to focus on the task at hand. Being fully present.

18. Optimism: an attitude reflecting hope. An ability to see the bright side. The belief in a favorable, positive outcome.

19. Patience: a lifelong spiritual practice. The capacity to accept or tolerate delay, trouble, or suffering without getting angry or upset. The ability to remain tolerant, to bear annoyance without complaint.

20. Perseverance: the willingness to fail, to do whatever it takes despite circumstances. To continue a course of action despite opposition. To persist against all odds. A quiet resilience.

21. Transparency: having a clear intention. The ability to communicate open and honestly. Operating in such a way that it is easy for others to see what actions are being performed.

22. Vision: the art of being able to see what hasn't materialized yet. The ability to look at the bigger picture and inspire others to dream. Insightful, intuitive, innovative, and imaginative.

23. Vulnerability: the willingness to risk exposure. Having the courage to show up and be seen.

We all have qualities that come more naturally to us and others that don't. So it's important to take the time to:

- Explore These Qualities: Which qualities do you resonate with the most? Which qualities could you improve upon to help strengthen your character?

- Recall These Qualities: Think of a challenging time when you may have used one or more of these qualities. How did these qualities come into play? What did you do? How did they help you?

- Apply These Qualities: Is there a way you could embody and then apply these qualities to your current situation? Which of these qualities could you draw upon the next time you feel depressed, stressed, or anxious?

Once you take the time to reflect on, integrate, and fully embody these qualities, your life will begin to transform.

So I invite you to get in the game, find your strength of character, your resilience. As Joseph P. Kennedy declared, "When the going gets tough, the tough get going." Remember, you have what it takes to move through this. Defeat is temporary and this too shall pass. Tomorrow is a new day, so stay committed and persistent in your efforts. Stay the course. Move through the fear, rise above adversity, and don't quit. Only from the ashes of who we once were can we rise up to become who we're meant to be.

So let the old you melt away as you rise up and out of the ashes of your former self. You have the spirit of perseverance running through you, and the sky's the limit!

CONCLUSION

"Whether you think you can, or you think you can't—you're right."
— HENRY FORD

We are not the sum of our past experiences, nor our current circumstances. We are the sum of our beliefs. Our beliefs dictate our life, for we perform at the level of our beliefs. What we believe drives what we do, and what we do determines our outcome. Our lives unfold based on the deep-seated beliefs that we hold. Our core belief systems shape our life and color our perceptions. Our overall health and happiness is affected by the way we think and feel. What we believe will either empower us or limit us. Therefore, we must be willing to challenge the beliefs we have about ourselves and others.

If we want to change our life, we must change our beliefs. We must reprogram our subconscious mind by removing the layers of programming that we adopted in childhood. Our behavior doesn't just deviate from its internal mapping—we can be sure we will sabotage anything that is out of alignment with our ingrained beliefs. We change our beliefs by changing our thoughts, by developing new habits, and by putting into place daily practices that encourage growth. We can overcome our resistance to change and harness the power of our beliefs by connecting to our higher self—the part of us that is already where we want to be—so that we can heal and manifest that which we say we want.

Right now, more than any time in history, we have the opportunity to reinvent ourselves, to redefine our identify. To open our eyes and see what must be done in order to shift through the lies, false beliefs, and judgments—and realign with our authentic selves. As a society, our capacity for dishonesty has grown out of proportion, and our ability to separate the truth from the lies seems, at times, to be next to impossible. This falsehood is shaking the core of our foundation both individually and collectively.

During this time of great uncertainty, let us bridge our divide and come together, for separation is merely an illusion. No matter where you are on the journey, if you're currently struggling in some way, shape, or form, know that you are not alone in the fight. The global impact of the coronavirus pandemic has left many of us unsure of how to cope with all the changes we are experiencing in both our personal and professional lives.

Through all the hardships we are now facing, one can only hope that this crisis has slowed us down enough to help us take a good look in the mirror. We can't always expect the truth from others, but we can expect it from ourselves. In the midst of all this chaos, we have an opportunity to unravel the web of deceit. To live a life of brave authenticity and vulnerability, a life in alignment with our true essence. That being said, we must be willing to embrace change—to get used to its many cycles of death and rebirth—to rise up and become stronger in spite of it all.

Change occurs on a collective level when a critical mass of people alter their perceptions and beliefs on how they want to live. Real change happens when we go above and beyond our words and noble intentions, when we put forth the effort and take action towards improving our lives. We cannot look to outside sources for our liberation. In order to find peace in this world, we must first find it within ourselves. We must be willing to do the inner work necessary for change to occur.

Let us not be prisoners of our past, nor slaves to our future. What once caused us pain can be transformed. We can break free from chains that bind us by resolving our generational trauma and developing a stronger sense of self. We can transform our trauma, from wounds to wisdom, through spiritual initiation. In order to move past our mass trauma, we must grow through it, experience it in all its glory so that we develop the skill sets necessary to fully thrive. The more we are tempered, the stronger we become. Our scars are proof of our spirit's courage. The unbreakable spirt that transcends circumstance.

We cannot control what's happening in the world, but we can control the part we play. We get to choose how we respond to and grow from our challenges. We can't change our past, but we can change our future, one present moment at a time. The obstacles on our path that we think are in our way, more often than not, lead us to unlocking our greatest potential. When we are able to tap into the power of resilience and choose to see setbacks as opportunities, we learn to bounce back more easily and readily from challenging times.

I hope this book has given you the ability to reflect and focus on what you can influence instead of focusing on what you have no control over. The road back to self is a journey. It doesn't happen overnight. It happens slowly but surely. With practice, your life will begin to change. Remember, everything happens for a reason and miracles happen every day, we just need to know where to look. You now have a roadmap to help you navigate through the storm. You have the tools you need to trust in the process, shift your perspective, push past your comfort zone, face your fears, challenge your beliefs, and reclaim your power. You have the strength to persevere, adapt, and pivot in order to make way for a brighter tomorrow.

They told me I was a failure, said you'll never succeed
A fool for believing, lost my will to achieve
Broken down and tired, how could this be
Not sure where to start, on the road, road back to me

Still searching for the answers, or so it seems
Picking up the pieces, of my shattered dreams
Putting together the puzzle, of who I'm meant to be
One step at a time, on the road, road back to me
It's time to move forward, and leave the past behind
Open up my heart and clear my mind

Expanding my horizons, looking deep inside
Painting a new picture, I can no longer hide
Breaking the chains that bind me, my spirit set free
Far and wide, on the road, road back to me

I'm on the road back, the road back, road back to me
I'm on the road back, the road back, road back to me

I'm on the road back, the road back, road back to me
I'm on the road back, the road back, road back to me

I'm on the road, oh I'm on my way back home
I'm on the road back, the road back, road back to me

"The Road Back To Me" by Adena Sampson

ACKNOWLEDGEMENTS

To My Family: My father, my mother, my two sisters, my brother-in-law, and niece and nephew. Thank you for all your love, light, and support. I love you dearly and I am blessed to share this journey with you.

To All My Soulmates (Friends & Lovers): Thank you for coming in to my life, mirroring me, and helping me grow.

To All My Mentors: Thank you for sharing your story, vulnerabilities, and insights so that I could in turn do the same.

To All My Earth Angels: You know who you are. Thank you for your belief, presence, and support during my darkest hours.

To God, the Universe, and All My Guides: Thank you for standing by me, having my back, protecting me, and guiding me in the right direction so that I may be of service and live a life on purpose.

WORKS CITED

"Ammonia: A Lyme Disease Exotoxin." *Tired of Lyme,* www. tiredoflyme.com/ammonia-a-lyme-disease-exotoxin.html.

Baker, Mitzi. "Undoing the Harm of Childhood Trauma and Adversity." *Undoing the Harm of Childhood Trauma and Adversity | UC San Francisco,* 11 June 2020, www.ucsf.edu/news/2016/10/404446/ undoing-harm-childhood-trauma-and-adversity.

Bransfield, Robert C. "Suicide and Lyme and Associated Diseases." *Neuropsychiatric Disease and Treatment,* Dove Medical Press, 16 June 2017, www.ncbi.nlm.nih.gov/pmc/articles/ PMC5481283/.

Forsgren, Scott, et al. "Mold and Mycotoxins: Often Overlooked Factors in Chronic Lyme Disease." *Hoffman Centre,* July 2014, hoffmancentre.com/wp-content/uploads/2016/12/Mold-and-Mycotoxins-Often-Overlooked-Factors-in-Chronic-Lyme-Disease.pdf.

Parish, Dana. "Lyme: The Infectious Disease Equivalent of Cancer, Says Top Duke Oncologist." *HuffPost,* HuffPost, 7 Dec. 2017, www. huffpost.com/entry/lyme-the-infectious-disea_b_9243460.

Rawls, Bill. "Epstein-Barr Virus: A Key Player in Chronic Illness." *RawlsMD,* 17 June 2019, rawlsmd.com/health-articles/ epstein-barr-virus-a-key-player-in-chronic-illness.

Shoemaker, Ritchie, et al. "Complement Split Products C3a and C4a Are Early Markers of Acute Lyme Disease in Tick Bite Patients in the United States." *International Archives of Allergy and Immunology*, 13 Feb. 2008, www.survivingmold.com/docs/Resources/Shoemaker%20Papers/Lyme_acute_C4a_1_08_glovsky.pdf.

"Should Lyme Disease Be Added to the Causes of Vocal Cord Paralysis?" *Daniel Cameron, MD, MPH*, CauseRoar, 20 Sept. 2019, www.danielcameronmd.com/lyme-disease-added-causes-vocal-cord-paralysis/.

"Treatment." *Centers for Disease Control and Prevention*, Centers for Disease Control and Prevention, 17 Dec. 2019, www.cdc.gov/lyme/treatment/index.html.

Treseler, Michelle. "Massachusetts in the Bull's-Eye; Proposed Lyme Disease Measure Could Save Lives." *LymeDisease.org*, 5 July 2016, www.lymedisease.org/ma-lyme-insurance-treseler/.

RESOURCES

As you are now aware, I spent the past twelve years fighting for my life. Western medicine wasn't cutting it, so I turned to alternative therapies/quantum healing and cutting-edge treatments/ technologies to fully heal. Having struggled so long with chronic illness, I do not endorse things lightly, as I refuse to give anyone false hope. I also feel it's my duty to speak up and share any and all resources that have helped me along my journey to recovery—if there's a possibility it can help support you and your loved ones, too—as it could very well be the piece of the puzzle that you've been searching for!

Testing

"Genes are like the story, and DNA is the language that the story is written in."
— SAM KEAN

23ANDME
DNA Genetic Testing & Analysis

23andMe is a privately held personal genomics and biotechnology company based in Sunnyvale, California. It is best known for providing a direct-to-consumer genetic testing service in which customers provide a saliva sample that is laboratory analyzed, using qualitative genotyping, to detect six variants in three genes in the DNA of adults for the purpose of reporting and interpreting information relating to the customer's genetic predispositions to health.

Contact 23AndMe INC: https://www.23andme.com
1-800-239-5230 | privacy@23andme.com
223 N. Mathilda Avenue, Sunnyvale, CA 94086, USA

IGeneX Inc.
Lyme Disease Testing | Tick-Borne Disease Testing

One of the main reasons why the CDC recommended two-tier ELISA/Western Blot tests are inconclusive, is that they aren't testing for the bacteria in the blood itself, but rather indirectly via antibody detection. Antibodies (proteins produced by the immune system in response to foreign invaders to help fight infection) take time to produce—which makes early detection hard to catch—and once produced, the antibodies can last for years making it difficult to gauge whether or not the infection has been resolved.

Another reason is that they are using outdated result criteria developed in 1994. A more comprehensive, up-to-date, and accurate form of testing is the IGeneX ImmunoBlot, which has a sensitivity rate nearly double that of the standard two-tier testing protocol. They test for more relevant strains of tick-borne disease and coinfections—as nearly one in four ticks carry more than one pathogen—to make up for the 25% of patients who are left undiagnosed due to faulty standard Lyme testing.

The IGeneX Advantage: For over 25 years, IGeneX has been the global leader in the research and development of tests that accurately detect Lyme disease, relapsing fever, and other tick-borne diseases. Tick-borne illnesses can affect every part of your life, and without effective diagnosis and treatment, symptoms can often worsen and progress into severe and even life-threatening health issues. And when you can't find the cause or a way to get better, your quality of life suffers. At IGeneX, we make it our singular mission to offer best-in-class testing for tick-borne diseases that delivers the most comprehensive and accurate results possible so you can find the right treatment path to restore your health and get back to enjoying your life.

Contact IgeneX: https://igenex.com

USA: 1-800-832-3200 | International: 1-650-424-1191

customerservice@igenex.com

556 Gibraltar Dr. Milpitas, CA 95035

Alternative Therapies

> *"Man's mind, once stretched by a new idea, never regains its original dimensions."*
> — OLIVER WENDELL HOLMES

DR. RONALD GREENAWALT - GREENAWALT CHIROPRACTIC

The Body Talk Method

Your body is designed to heal itself. When all the parts and systems of the body com'municate with each other, healing happens naturally. However, stress can cause communication breakdowns, resulting in discomfort and disease. BodyTalk identifies these breakdowns and uses a light tapping technique to restore communication, helping the body to heal itself. Conditions that typically improve with BodyTalk:

- Allergies

- Depression

- Headaches/Migraines

- Back Pain

- Insomnia

- Stress/Anxiety

- Sports Performance

- Arthritis

Dr. Ronald Greenawalt approaches his patients with awareness that every individual possesses distinct differences and needs even when presenting similar complaints. He supports open communication, which aids him in discovering the key contributing factors of the person's particular illness or wellness goals in order to formulate an individual treatment plan to best benefit the patient.

Dr. Greenawalt's pursuit is to bridge Eastern and Western medicine, bringing a new level of physical consciousness to the community. He utilizes applied kinesiology as an adjunct to gentle spinal adjusting, as well as other modalities, as its shown to be an effective holistic way of treating and obtaining desired results.

Dr. Greenawalt believes that conservative treatment like chiropractic should always be our first health approach. He believes in an interdisciplinary approach to resolving health challenges when applicable. Allopathic medicine and chiropractic work well together when the patient's condition and recovery is first and foremost in caring for their needs.

Dr. Greenawalt has been an absolute angel in my life! My body has always responded well to chiropractic care, as there is a definite link between the alignment of the vertebrae and the body's ability to function properly, including strengthening of the immune system. More importantly, the BodyTalk method helps us get down to the root cause of many of our ailments—by tapping into our subconscious mind and becoming aware of the limiting beliefs we hold—so that we can reprogram them.

Contact Greenawalt Chiropractic: https://greenawaltchirolv.com
702-363-8989 | greenawalt.chiropractic@gmail.com
7500 West Sahara Avenue Las Vegas, NV 89117

DR. ANTHONY SMITH - LYMESTOP
Natural Treatment for Lyme Disease

A dramatic breakthrough in the evaluation and treatment of Lyme disease. Dr. Anthony Smith is featured in the book *New Paradigms in Lyme Disease Treatment: 10 Top Doctors Reveal Healing Strategies that Work*. During his thirty-eight years as a natural health care provider, Dr. Smith has pioneered numerous effective healing techniques including AllerTouch, the CranioBiotic Technique (CBT), and a CBT-based muscle rejuvenation technique called MyoBiotix.

In early 2009, he was shocked to learn that his own chronic, frustrating symptoms had one insidious cause—Lyme disease.

Dr. Smith was determined to find a cure, discovering that the best therapeutic outcomes were achieved with magnetic stimulation—BioMagnetic Lyme Points (BLPs). This revolutionary therapy has been a Godsend for many who have suffered with this debilitating disease.

Enthusiastic reports of LymeStop's effectiveness spread quickly and Dr. Smith was honored to be the Lyme literate doctor for people throughout the United States and numerous other countries. Whether you've just been diagnosed, or have already "tried everything," we urge you to experience the extraordinary healing power of LymeStop.

Dr. Tony played an integral role in my recovery and healing. I was at what I thought was my end when I found LymeStop. I had tried next to everything with no success and within minutes of my first visit I could feel his treatment working. He was able to pinpoint a long list of bacterial, viral, and fungal coinfections—along with a few key cofactors—that were the underlying cause of my suffering. He is known to have a very high success rate treating patients that fly in to see him from all over the world as a last resort. If you are suffering in any way, shape, or form with any deemed "mystery illness," I highly suggest working with Dr. Tony!

Contact Dynamic Health: http://lymestop.com
208-765-8061 | dhealth@frontier.com
2065 Riverstone Dr. Suite 102 Coeur D'Alene, ID 83814

LOW DOSE NALTREXONE
Immune System Regulator

Low Dose Naltrexone (LDN) is being used as a regulator of the immune system, providing relief to patients with autoimmune diseases and central nervous system disorders. Whilst it is not licensed by the FDA specifically for these conditions, physicians are permitted to prescribe LDN "off-label" for treatments they think are appropriate.

The apparently diverse conditions in which LDN appears to have a therapeutic effect are united by their ability to benefit from increased levels of endorphins. Examples of the successful use of LDN, supported by studies as well as reported by patients to date, include the following conditions:

- Autoimmune disorders

- Cancer

- Chronic pain

- Crohn's disease

- Depression

- Dissociative disorder

- Fibromyalgia

- Gulf War illness

- HIV

- IBS

- Lyme disease

- Multiple sclerosis (MS)

- Parkinson's

- Psychiatric conditions

- PTSD

- Ulcerative colitis, and more...

LDN has noticeably strengthened my immune system and lessened my body's inflammation, making a big difference in my overall health. Recent studies have also shown LDN to be a potential therapeutic candidate for COVID-19. Please consult your physician for more details and visit: https://www.ldnscience.org

Cutting-Edge Treatments & Technologies

"We are finally entering an exciting time in medicine where we have the technology to custom-tailor treatment and preventive protocols just as we'd custom-tailor a suit or designer gown to one's individual body."
— DAVID AGUS

DR. JOHN CATANZARO - NEO7LOGIX
Precision Bio-Science

A unique and truly personalized approach to activate and regulate your immune system to defeat disease. Every individual is unique. Even if two people share a disease with the same name, these can be two entirely different disease processes whose only commonality is the name.

We at Neo7Logix analyze each patient's immune system to find the immunological problems that have allowed the disease process to occur. After testing and analysis, we identify where the immune system is weak and develop the precise mix of peptides that work to bring the body back to health.

Neo7Logix develops personalized immune therapy using a patient's individualized genetic, cell, molecular protein data and creates a "best fit" immunomolecular programming also known as PBIMA (Precision-Based ImmunoMolecular Augmentation). Neo7Logix has recently completed a preclinical study that demonstrated greater than 99% reduction of viral load in mice infected with mutant coronavirus HCoV-229E using anti-HCoV-229E (COVID-19) PBIMA-SOLVx with no adverse effects.

Next-generation sequencing (NGS) is the future of DNA research and health care; the applications of this technology have the potential to enhance individualized patient care. Costs are coming down, and the rate at which we are able to sequence DNA is rapidly increasing, which makes cutting-edge technology accessible to more researchers and clinicians. This sophisticated sequencing method is helping us better understand how the expression of genetic variants affects us. For example, NGS allows scientists to more easily identify exome mutations, which are thought to contain the vast majority of mutations that lead to human diseases. With NGS, we can efficiently compare the DNA of thousands of people and explore the individual genes that cause conditions such as cancer, viral-related disease and infection, autoimmune disease, neurodegenerative disease, schizophrenia, autism, and regenerative health.

Dr. John A. Catanzaro, NMD, Neo7Logix Founder & CEO, received his Doctorate of Naturopathic Medicine from Bastyr University in 1995. He has retired from clinical practice and was the former founder and CEO of the largest integrative cancer center in Seattle. He innovated patient-precision patient matched immuno-peptides and cell therapy to train defense cells to eradicate very advanced cancers considered incurable failing all conventional treatments with successful outcomes. He also was affiliate/adjunct faculty for Bastyr University and taught integrative cancer outpatient medicine to medical students and resident physicians for fifteen years.

He served on the Bastyr Institutional Review Board for six years. He was appointed by the governor and served Washington Department of Health Quality Assurance Board for naturopathic medicine for five years as Co-Chair. He also served on the CDC Medical Board Cancer Commission representing Washington state for two years as a medical advisor on integrative cancer care. Dr. Catanzaro also was a former member of the American Association for Cancer Research (AACR).

Dr. John is a brilliant mind specializing in genetics, epigenetics, and personalized medicine. I first met Dr. John when I needed my 23andMe genetic data analyzed. We discussed the many underlying genetic components and the role they played in my recovery, and I was put on a health plan to address these issues accordingly. The support and education I got when working with Dr. John was second to none! If anyone is seeking an integrative, cutting-edge approach to address chronic disease or COVID-19, I highly recommend getting in touch with Neo7Logix and the work that they are doing.

Contact Neo7Logix LLC: https://neo7logix.com
206-718-5467 | info@neo7logix.com
539 W. Commerce St. #2886 Dallas, TX 785208

THE HEALY
Frequencies for Life

The Healy is an FDA-cleared class II medical device. It's a wearable micro-current technology that supports the endocannabinoid system and boosts the powerhouse of our cells—our mitochondria—by increasing ATP levels. This device scans your energetic field and then delivers specific individualized frequencies to your body to help address any issue that you'd like to improve.

These frequencies help with everything from arthritis to neuropathy, from nutrition to vitamin supplementation, from balancing hormones to helping you sleep, as well as the ability to kill viruses, protozoans, fungi, bacteria, etc. It's recommended for anyone currently dealing with chronic pain, inflammation, or illness, and all the biohackers and health-conscious, performance-based types out there who share a vision of vibrant health and who are committed to being part of the solution for a better tomorrow.

The Healy has been a great tool for me to use to manage any overwhelm, anxiety, depression, inflammation, and other painful aches and symptoms that arise, in particular with the use of the Healy Resonance, which works on a more subtle quantum physic level to harmonize our own bioenergetics. Having access to this type of medical technology at home and at such a low cost has been a Godsend. I wish I had access to this earlier on in my journey. Highly recommended!

For more information or to schedule a resonance session contact: lvloud@gmail.com
https://www.healy.shop/en/partner/?partnername=LVLOUD

Quantum & Frequency Healing

"If you want to find the secrets of the universe, think in terms of energy, frequency, and vibration."
— NIKOLA TESLA

CHRIS FABISH - TRULY HOLISTIC
Health Consultancy

Chris Fabish is a nurse with twelve years' experience in the medical field and holds a post-graduate certification in nutrition. He uses the True Quantum Healing (TQH) method to find out the real causes to your health problems. His goal is to find the underlying causes of disease and work alongside you to remove your health problem, not just the symptoms!

For example, if your complaint is diabetes, this method will find out the root cause (stressor). This may be a virus, parasite, bacterial infection, or negative energy. Once he finds what the stressor is and where in the body it is, he uses crystalline energy tools to neutralize (remove) the stressor. The TQH method allows him to work on conditions such as:

- Cancer

- Heart disease, including arrhythmias, blood pressure problems, and coagulation issues

- Asthma/COPD

- Eczema, dermatitis, other skin conditions

- Spinal vertebrae and disc misalignment, arthritis and joint misalignment

- Diabetes, types 1 and 2

- Autoimmune disorders such as rheumatoid arthritis, Crohn's disease, ulcerative colitis, etc.

- Addiction and mental illnesses such as depression, anxiety, and soul fragmentation

- Negative energies, entities, spiritual attachments

- Gastrointestinal issues such as obstructions and blockages

- Removing stubborn cold and flu-like symptoms, and much more...

Thank God I was led to Chris. I started noticing a shift in my overall health right away after only a couple sessions. Within twenty-four hours, I experienced a major shift in my energy! I went from having chronic fatigue to a bounce in my step and a shift even in my voice. The people closest to me started to notice. There were days I didn't have to take my regular nap and I was able to run multiple errands on my own, which is unheard of. So many of the chronic symptoms that plagued my days have been lightened tremendously or lifted altogether. Nothing short of a miracle! I highly recommend Chris and am confident he can help get to the root of your health issues, whatever they may be. When all else fails, you must be willing to do whatever it takes! Thank you, Chris, there are no words to truly describe my deepest gratitude.

Contact Truly Holistic: http://trulyholistic.net
021857885 | chrisfabish@hotmail.com
19 Hori street, Brooklands, New Plymouth 4310, NZ

Advanced Cell Training
A Holistic Program

Advanced Cell Training (ACT) is a holistic home-based program that trains the body to recognize cellular behaviors that cause symptoms and corrects the behaviors by resetting the body's biological response to pathogens, toxins, allergens, and trauma.

Maybe you have been ill for many years and spent thousands of dollars seeing doctors and specialists only to fall into an endless cycle of relief and relapse. Perhaps you've realized that doctors may have helped you, but they haven't been able to heal you. Now you are seeking to try something different, something that delivers better and lasting results.

Our clients have trained their bodies to overcome chronic Lyme disease, multiple sclerosis, fibromyalgia, rheumatoid arthritis, lupus, chronic fatigue syndrome, depression, anxiety, asthma, allergies, insomnia, migraines, panic attacks, PTSD, Crohn's disease, seizures, OCD, addiction, eczema, and much more! Can you imagine a life without pain and sickness?

Contact Advance Cell Training:

https://www.advancedcelltraining.com

support@advancedcelltraining.com

1050 Main Street Unit 17, East Greenwich, RI 02818

ABOUT THE AUTHOR

Adena Sampson M.Sc., Founder of Outloud Productions & The Unbreakable Spirit Movement, is a Breakthrough Coach, Inspirational Speaker, Singer-Songwriter, and Best-Selling Author. Having overcome the insurmountable, Adena leads by example, teaching us how to turn challenges into victories and inspiring us to live a more authentic, courageous, and passionate life!

A gifted speaker, emcee, narrator, and presenter, from workshops and seminars, voiceovers and jingles, to commercials and broadcasting, Adena has offered extraordinary customer service and representation for many professional associations, including a number of Fortune 500 companies.

An entrepreneur at heart, Adena has an extensive background in event management, media, marketing, and sales and has built and trained solid teams. Adena made her mark in the network marketing industry as a high performance leader with an online technology company, ranking in the top 40 of 20,000, and was responsible for the growth and expansion of over 500 affiliates.

As an accomplished singer-songwriter, guitarist, and producer, Adena has graced the stage across the globe and has had the opportunity to open up for Patti LaBelle, Wayne Newton, Jim Brickman, Nils Lofgren, and more. She's a born traveler with a love for adventure and a passion for life, a woman that sings from her soul with a gritty raw power and passion rarely heard today.

No matter the medium, with her vibrant energy, radiant smile, and engaging sense of humor, Adena is sure to add color to your event!

For more information please visit: *www.AdenaSampson.com*

PAY IT FORWARD

Love this book? Don't forget to leave a review!

Every review matters and makes a difference.

So head on over to Amazon, or wherever you purchased this

book, to leave a review and spread the love.

Thank you kindly.

WHAT'S YOUR STORY?

I'd like to invite you to share your own story of how you overcame the insurmountable. Please visit www.theunbreakablespirit.com to submit your story and join the community.

If you are still navigating through the storm, you will be able to access other resources such as weekly blogs, podcasts, social media handles, and connect with others who are going through and/or have gone through much of the same.

It is my hope that this inspiring group of "unbreakable spirits" can help you realize that you are not alone on this journey and that you have the ability, against all odds, to make it through!

CPSIA information can be obtained
at www.ICGtesting.com
Printed in the USA
LVHW042051160723
752571LV00026B/24/J